EMPOWERED EATING

Binge Free Forever

KIM STEVENSON FARMAKIS

First published by Ultimate World Publishing 2020
Copyright © 2020 Kim Stevenson Farmakis

ISBN

Paperback - 978-1-922372-10-9
Ebook - 978-1-922372-11-6

Kim Stevenson Farmakis has asserted her right under the Copyright, Designs and Patents Act 1988 to be identified as the author of this work. The information in this book is based on the author's experiences and opinions. The publisher specifically disclaims responsibility for any adverse consequences, which may result from use of the information contained herein. Permission to use information has been sought by the author. Any breaches will be rectified in further editions of the book.

All rights reserved. No part of this publication may be reproduced, stored in or introduced into a retrieval system, or transmitted in any form, or by any means (electronic, mechanical, photocopying, recording or otherwise) without the prior written permission of the author. Any person who does any unauthorised act in relation to this publication may be liable to criminal prosecution and civil claims for damages. Enquiries should be made through the publisher.

Cover design: Ultimate World Publishing
Layout and typesetting: Ultimate World Publishing
Editor: Marinda Wilkinson

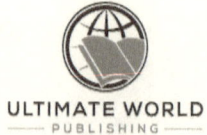

Ultimate World Publishing
Diamond Creek,
Victoria Australia 3089
www.writeabook.com.au

Testimonials

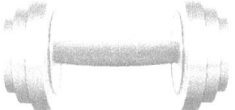

I began my journey as a client of Kim, in hope and in search of a healthy, happy and balanced life, physically, emotionally and holistically. I could never have foreseen the leaps and bounds I have since made in my personal life as a result of working with Kim.

For many, many years, I sought psychological therapy, natural and pharmaceutical treatments, to try and find balance and healing. Countless therapy sessions and heavy financial outlays with psychologists and psychiatrists failed to identify the issue – yet Kim found what I truly needed to work on in only a few short sessions of her personalised life coaching. This was something that all the psychotherapists and medications could never pinpoint or treat in all of my clinical history, ever. Through the healing of my emotional being, my physical health has improved immeasurably!

There is a raw, genuine truth and beauty in Kim. Her honesty, understanding and nurturing of the soul will help you to physically and spiritually connect both back to one whole being again. Through Kim, I found my truth. I am eternally grateful for the privilege of being coached and mentored by Kim. My life is now always moving forward and growing each day, little by little, achieving unforeseen and great things.

T. Moran

When I first heard about Kim and her emotional eating strategies, I was in a vicious cycle of fasting and overeating. I was miserable, and had steadily regained 50kgs that I'd worked so hard to lose a few years earlier. I bought a ticket to Kim's next workshop as a last-ditch attempt to do something about my health but I didn't go because I hated myself after bingeing the night before. When Kim reached out to me a week later, offering me a free ticket to her next workshop, I grasped that lifeline gratefully. Kim's gesture of kindness gave me the courage to attend the next workshop. Attending it transformed my life.

Over a period of 12 months, I applied Kim's emotional eating strategies to every aspect of my life. I started small, buying myself a water bottle for my desk at work. I found myself packing healthy lunches and, to my amazement, eating more food. Working with Kim, I committed to changing my self-talk from critical to compassionate. I stopped avoiding mirrors and started to love myself. I learned that good nutrition, regular exercise and improved sleep combined to give me the energy to take part in activities that I enjoyed. I rediscovered what Kim calls my 'x-factor' and started to have fun again. I can honestly say that I'm a happier and healthier person as a result.

If you're looking to develop a healthy relationship with food, I thoroughly recommend following Kim's emotional eating strategies. They will transform your life.

K. Creaner

Kim's coaching is different to other professionals I have seen. Her sessions are like unfolding the layers of an onion, she will keep pulling at the layers until the truth reveals itself, whilst providing strategies and homework for the healing to begin.

S. Mackay

At 37 years of age I have seen more therapists, counsellors, hypnotherapists, and psychologists then most people have had hot dinners. After only two sessions with Kim, I have finally gained the insights, understanding – and most importantly, the tools – to move forward with life and be truly at peace with where I want to be. I can be completely honest to say what I feel from a safe space, knowing I will be challenged to grow. If you have anything holding you back in life, this woman is the one to help you break down your shaky structures and rebuild a solid foundation. I cannot recommend Kim highly enough.

If you do anything for yourself, let it be under the amazing guidance and introspective journey that is Kim's own personal approach. Caring and nurturing whilst challenging you to be the best version of you! Bring on the rest of the adventure because for the first time ever, I'm excited to discover more about the whys, and in turn, change the direction of where.

S. Holmes

Kim conspires with you to slay the dragons disguised as the limiting behaviours stopping you reaching your fitness and health goals. Dragon slaying with Kim is fun and when you step back and see just how far you have come with her guidance and support you can't help but feel stronger, more confident and accomplished.

A. Condie

Through food coaching with Kim, I now have no more guilt around food. I'm eating more food than I've ever eaten before and maintaining my body weight. As an active female it can be hard eating what others think is a lot of food, and the perceived judgement associated with this. First of all Kim gave me permission to eat more. Over time working with Kim I have gained the knowledge and tools to think rationally about my diet. I need this amount of food to be my best in my training and to perform in my everyday life. I no longer feel judged by others (which of course was entirely in my own head). By taking the guilt away from food I actually don't even want to eat junk food anymore.

Through life coaching with Kim I have investigated what I value in life. I now feel I have more time in my day as I spend it working on or towards the things I love. I feel more energised in all aspects of my life as I'm not living in a way that's incongruent with my values.

My relationships are better because I can verbalise what it is I want from the relationship, but I also have the tools to help those I care for work towards their goals. I can hear others with different values and discuss their difference of opinion without taking it personally. I know that those who love me want only what's best for me and if I can verbalise what that is then we can work towards this together.

I actually have work goals now. Previously my goals were all health and fitness related. Before life coaching with Kim I never even wanted to work towards the next tier in my career. I was happy to just stay put. Now the idea of progressing in my career is exciting to me. I always felt my life lacked balance, but with Kim's help I'm now working towards a more complete and fulfilled version of me.

E. Padovan

I don't know how Kim did it, but with her amazing coaching she got down into the scary thing called my head! I swear she had to climb over a rainbow, jump across cotton candy puffs and got stuck in unicorn poo – but she made it out the other side and got me there with her. There were tears, I won't lie. Sorry if the graphics scare some people but this wouldn't be a true reference if it wasn't the real me, because I love me now, and all I have to offer!

So I had this plan, to try this business, but kept putting it off because I wasn't 'ready yet'. After glorious coaching I found what I was looking for, I found me, I found my values, I found what meant most to me – and in doing all this, I realised what I wanted to do, and remembered who I was. I realised that what I wanted to do I already knew – I had already experienced it in past years, just never as a business.

Now two months into my new venture, business is beaming – and why? Because I have a confidence I have never had, well not as far as I could remember anyhow. I have an understanding that there's more to me than just being the 'good one' – now I'm the 'Damn Good At It One'. Hee heee, Kim pulled that confidence out of me, taught me how to find it and taught me how to use it. The journey I needed was not that of losing weight, but a journey into my mind to find me and find my happy, and fitness was an extra bonus! My mind is so clear I take things in, I learn and I build – my head had been foggy for too long. Now it's clear and I'm on fire, it's crazy but it's amazing! Life couldn't be better with a healthy, happy, successful me. Thank you Kim Stevenson you superstar you!

Crystalina The Great

I have only recently started working with Kim, and within a short period of time, she has allowed me to be comfortable with my body and the way I look, be proud of my assets and be ok with my flaws. The conversations we have are real and honest, something I have struggled to do many times before. I am really excited to see how much I can grow with Kim, as up until now I haven't felt ready to love myself as who I am, and have avoided taking care of myself, and treating myself the way I deserve to be treated. Now, I have started to learn the value of my body, and how to focus on what it can do, not what it can't. A very valuable lesson which I can't wait to explore further. It's all thanks to Kim.

S. Keetman

After years of yo-yo dieting I started to dig into what was going on in my mind. With Kim's coaching and support I've challenged and reset my beliefs to create a new and sustainable mindset, my new normal. Pulling your stories apart and rebuilding them can be confronting, but I'd highly recommend it as the key to succeeding, not just in relation to health and fitness, but in so many areas of your life.

Sharyn

I can't thank Kim enough. She is kind, passionate and truly cares for her clients. I started working with Kim at a point in my life where it felt like everything was falling apart. She provided support, guidance and asked the tough questions. Now, I have not only been able to get my nutrition and fitness back on track, but my mindset around life as a whole has also improved drastically. She is amazing and I highly recommend her.

D. Beaudreau

Kim is a wonderfully positive, supportive and practical coach. Her mindset training has been invaluable. I highly recommend her services whatever it is you're trying to achieve.

C. Halloran

Kim has taught me to identify and practically apply routines and rituals into my day that help set my mindset up for success. By using the tools Kim has taught me about rituals and managing my state, I feel more positive and in control of my emotions, and am better able to choose resourceful ways to respond to challenges rather than bingeing on chocolate.

Jennine

Mindset is to success just as diet is to exercise – 80% mental and 20% action. This is what I constantly tell myself. You must 'feed' your brain positivity just as you feed your body a proper diet to get optimum results. Kim has helped with both as she combines both mental and physical coaching. Mindset trumps skill set any day of the week and success is an inside job!

C. Neist

Dedication

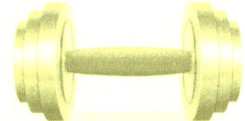

To my husband Billy, thank you for showing me true love and supporting all my crazy dreams.

To my Mum, who taught me to be strong and independent.

To Joe, my powerlifting coach who took me all the way to the top. We still have a lot to achieve.

To Cath, for igniting my love and passion for business.

To God, for giving me the gift to help others.

To my friends and family who have been there when I need.

Contents

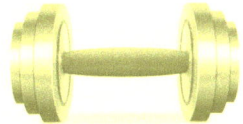

Testimonials iii
Dedication xi
Introduction xv
Chapter 1: Making it happen 1
Chapter 2: The salad is greener 15
Chapter 3: What really matters? 29
Chapter 4: Owning you 43
Chapter 5: Sexy and confident 55
Chapter 6: Blame elegantly 71
Chapter 7: CAR and STONE 79
Chapter 8: It's not food, it's me 91
Chapter 9: Life detox 101
Chapter 10: Strawberry friends and
    chocolate friends 111
Chapter 11: You are a shero 119
Chapter 12: Piranha to nirvana 133
Afterword 143
About the Author 145
Acknowledgements 149

Introduction

If you've ever eaten your emotions, raided the pantry when you're stressed, found yourself bored and looking for something interesting in the fridge or have finished the whole packet of Tim Tams without even realising it – this book is for you.

If you've tried so many diets but still find yourself yo-yoing. If you turn to food as a reward. If you use it as a pick-me-up when you have had a bad day, a fight with your partner, the kids are driving you mad or your boyfriend dumps you.

You are not alone – and it's shame, fear, past stories and emotions that keep you going back to the pantry.

Since 2006, I've helped women in the fitness industry to eat well and exercise. However, many kept sabotaging their results. It wasn't from a lack of knowledge about what to eat or pushing hard enough in training. It was their mindset and beliefs about self that kept them on the roller-coaster of emotional eating. So I studied life coaching, NLP and high-performance coaching to better support them — and in this book, I want to share my knowledge, insights and tried and tested techniques with you.

Empowered Eating is designed to be your best friend on the journey to healing your relationship with food. The unsexy part is, that it is going to take some emotional work — but really, the unsexiest part to any transformation is always the work.

Are you ready to change? Are you ready to do the work? Yes! All we need is an hour a week together. If an hour is too much, find 10 minutes and do one of the easiest activities first. There is no correct order, there is no right or wrong. You are the expert in your life. I am here as your support. The tiniest step will get the ball rolling. One of my favourite sayings is, 'How do you eat an elephant? One spoonful at a time'. Eat that one, tiny, itty-bitty spoonful today.

Once you have set aside time for yourself every week (because you are worthy of this time), invest in a journal. It can be an exercise book, leather bound or something from kikki.K, just make sure it feels special to you. I even go as far as having a special purple pen for my journals. This journal is precious as there will be insights, breakthroughs and practical tools that you will develop along the way that are unique to you.

I would also suggest having a favourite spot that you would like to do the work. This creates a positive anchor to your growth and development. It could be a beanbag, a place in the garden, on the floor (tummy time is really playful and fun), your bed, the ocean (just don't use that as a roadblock not to do the work because you can't get there), a park or an oval. Anywhere you can create calm.

Now that you are all set, pick a chapter to read. There is a sequence to the chapters, however, if a chapter is calling you, go there first.

At the end of each chapter there will be activities to do. I call these your Empowered Eating Toolbox. I will ask some thought-provoking

INTRODUCTION

questions and give you ideas to implement a strategy that WILL work. You can tweak this strategy to make it your own – don't forget that you are the expert in your life.

I love hearing your wins and breakthroughs. Tag me on Instagram or Facebook and use the hashtag #EmpoweredEatingMindset.

- https://www.facebook.com/Transformations-by-Kim-234947206582487/
- https://www.instagram.com/kim.stevenson.farmakis
- https://www.linkedin.com/in/kim-stevenson-farmakis-2b6b68bb
- https://transformationsbykim.com/home

Chapter 1

Making it happen

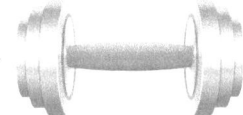

If my reason isn't big enough, my excuses will be. If you have a big enough why, you will find the how.
					Tony Robbins

We've all been there. It's been a bad day. You feel like crap and nothing seems to go right. You just want to go home and smash that bottle of wine or eat some chocolate. Heck, why stop there, you want the whole block!

But what stops you? *Knowing your why.*

Having a big enough why is the emotional driver that you need to get out of bed in the morning to train, or to not drink that whole bottle of wine after work. *When you have a big enough why the how will take care of itself.*

As my favourite guru Tony Robbins said, 'As human beings we move towards pleasure and away from pain'. By identifying your big reason why you create that emotional pull you need when you are lacking motivation.

Living in Canberra at the start of my health and fitness journey many years ago it was very challenging to get out of bed in the morning because it was freezing cold. One of my emotional drivers was to fit into a size 12 Jacqui E pants. As a way of motivating myself I decided to hang these pants on my wardrobe door which I saw when I opened my eyes in the morning. Most of the time it worked because it reminded me visually of what I was working towards. At the time I was a size 16 and had really unhealthy behaviours around food and couldn't motivate myself to train. I know this is hard to believe considering I'm now a size 8 and an international athlete who says training is like breathing! From a neuroscience perspective this worked in many ways as it gave me the visual anchor that activated my reticular activating system (RAS) in my brain and created stronger neurological pathways towards the healthy habit. Throughout this book we are going to use your RAS as a superpower.

Your RAS is a bunch of nerves at your brainstem that filters out unnecessary information so the important information gets through. Think of your RAS as a nightclub bouncer that works for your brain. It makes sure your brain doesn't become overcrowded with more information than it can handle.

Why do we need this bouncer? Well, your senses are constantly feeding so much information to your brain that you can't possibly pay attention to all of it. The RAS never gets a break! Our senses take in 10,000 pieces of information every second. So that we don't become overloaded we need to delete, distort and generalise information. It also associates things together to take short cuts. If I say salt, you automatically think pepper.

You may associate fun with the beach or movies with popcorn. Some of these associations run deep from childhood. Some may be serving you well – while others may not. Breaking the unhelpful neurological pathways will take work.

Another example of your RAS at work is if you are thinking of buying a BMW. Suddenly, you will see them everywhere. It's not that people went out and purchased more BMWs, it's that your RAS is in overdrive deleting and distorting all other cars on the road to help you focus on what you want.

So let's use your RAS as a superpower to work towards what you want. Once you have completed this exercise you are going to find something physical (your anchor) to remind yourself of your goal, like I did with those size 12 Jacquie E pants.

Discovering your why

I can testify that you need to have your big reason why to create new and stronger neurological pathways towards new behaviours. As the saying goes, motivation gets you started but habit keeps you going. We are going to use your visual anchors and your big reason why to get you motivated and form habits that lead you towards your new goals.

To create this anchor we need to find your big reason why. One of the Toolbox strategies for this chapter is to create a list of 30 reasons why you want to achieve your goals. The first few will be really easy, and then I am going to push you for your 30. This is where the magic happens because you start to dig into your emotional drivers. These are your big reasons why. After listing all your reasons why, we can then identify what would be an anchor for you.

One summer I was going home to my family in Noosa and was needing motivation to be more focused with my nutrition and training. When doing my big reason why list it came down to being confident on the beach with my brothers and saying yes to everything while on holidays. Like me, many of my clients check out of social situations and fun activities because they feel self-conscious and fat. My big reasons why list revealed that I didn't want to miss out on fun activities with my brothers. From this list I was able to create an anchor of hanging my bikini top on my pantry door so that I could see it and it was my visual reminder to my big reason why which was to have fun on the beach with my brothers.

Your big reason why and anchor will help in those times of temptation. Along this journey you will be challenged by your friends. The ability to confidently say no and stand in your space will come from having your big reason why. If you're brave enough you could even share it with them. The more you share your dreams the more support you will get.

The biggest excuse most people say is that they lack motivation. It's not motivation that's the problem; it's the emotional pull towards your goal.

If you have an important goal, it needs a big why. Without it, you will lack the determination and resolve you need to overcome the challenges you'll inevitably encounter along the path to achieving it.

Most people focus almost completely on the how and in the process, they miss the all-important *why*. Have you found your why? When it comes to your goals, if you're uninspired and not making the progress you'd like, look more deeply to uncover your most important and meaningful reasons why.

Empowered Eating story time

As an athlete having a big enough why can impact so many little things. Since 2010 I have competed in bodybuilding at a national level and represented Australia at an international level for powerlifting. My big reason why was to always do my best at an athletic level. This means that I only drink a handful of times a year and have a two-glass limit, as that impacts my testosterone levels, which as a female I want to get as much as I can to lift the most amount of weight. Females biologically have a naturally lower amount of testosterone and we need to work harder to have the same gains as the guys.

Whenever I travel I always take my food with me, because it's important that I get the most nutritionally dense food that I can and adhere to my protein and fibre targets. I'm also coeliac which takes away the easy option. I often hear clients come to me with various different excuses why they couldn't eat healthy while they travelled. If they were coeliac and had no other option they would choose something healthy. They simply couldn't settle for McDonalds because it was easy. Being coeliac and having my big enough why means that I have to be a lot more prepared.

Having a big enough why to represent our country meant that self-care also took precedence. I will take time out to do yoga, go to the beach, read and have downtime because if I am overly stressed it impacts my ability to lift. Having a big enough why means I go to bed at a reasonable hour instead of staying up all hours. Sleep is so important for recovery.

Another layer to my big reason why is to make my brothers proud of me and lead by example that anything is possible. I will push my body to take it to the next level. I want them to see that anything is possible if you put your mind to it.

Being an athlete and a business owner means that I need to be ultra-organised. My reason why is to impact the world and change people's lives, but to balance it with family commitments, running a house and general life admin means that I have to be ultra-organised. This is the reason why every Sunday I sit down and plan out my whole entire week so that I can ensure that everything fits. Training is allocated first so that I can maximise the time that I have the most amount of energy and is reflective of my biggest goal.

They may seem like little things, however, all these little tiny things add up to ensure that I show up the best I can in my dual profession as an athlete and a businesswoman. I need energy to run a house, while spending time with my Greek family. When you have a big enough reason why, the how will take care of itself. I don't question going to bed early or training because my why is big enough.

If you are looking for a big enough why to do weight training I can testify from training women since 2006 that when you become physically stronger, it has a flow on effect to your mental and emotional strength. Your posture improves which means you face the world differently. You have the confidence to stand in your space and discover your inner strength, so you can tackle anything that life throws at you.

Therese's story

After Therese did her 30 big reasons, she discovered the following three were her most important 'whys' for being fit and healthy.

1) Increase in energy

I want to be able to play outside with my son again. He's a very active eight-year-old and I couldn't shoot hoops with him without losing my breath.

This is a massive reason why that has an emotional pull from her son. To be able to play with him and not miss out on these precious moments to create memories.

The anchor: A picture of her son as a screensaver.

2) Outlet

I have a super stressful job running a business with my sister. We almost dissolved the business because I snapped over a proposal we were writing. I was just so stressed and had pent-up anger. One of the ways I use to de-stress from uni is to go for a run.

Relationships are so important to nurture and it is our responsibility is to show up the best that we can. One way that Therese can do that is to make sure she has her outlet of running, as this is her way of de-stressing, reducing cortisol and not snapping at her sister. Her big reason why is to nurture her relationship with her sister and keep the business in flow, which is her only income.

The anchor: A keychain on her gym bag with a pic of her and her sister when they were teenagers at a family holiday and another keyring of the business logo.

3) Feel good in my own skin again

My husband thinks I'm still the goddess I was when we first met 19 years ago, but I can't see it just yet. I know he deserves the best of me, the me that used to be confident, happy and felt sexy when we first met.

Sometimes we are driven to do things more for other people than we are ourselves. You have permission to use this as emotional leverage (your why) to get you started. For Therese to do this for her husband was a bigger pull than doing it for herself, she wanted to feel inside what he saw. To do this she needed to train and eat healthy. When you eat well it has a massive impact on how you feel. Good quality nutritious food makes you feel good and radiate your goddess factor.

Anchor: Changing her passwords to 'I am a Goddess'.

Activity

Step 1: Take out your favourite pen, and in the space below (or your journal if you wish) list 30 reasons why you want to achieve your goal.

1) _____

2) _____

3) _____

4) _____

5) _____

6) _____

7) _____

8) _____

9) _____

10) _____

11) _____

12) _____

MAKING IT HAPPEN

13) _____

14) _____

15) _____

16) _____

17) _____

18) _____

19) _____

20) _____

21) _____

22) _____

23) _____

24) _____

25) _____

26) _____

27) _____

28) _____

29) _____

30) _____

Step 2: Look closely at the recurring themes in your list to uncover your big why. The first few reasons that you give are going to be from your logical brain. When you ask yourself a few more times (or 30 times like above) you will eventually discover your unconscious reason why. That's where the real magic is. This is the emotional buy-in that you need to leverage change. Sometimes these emotional buy-ins are reflective of our goals. My husband really wants to build a race car to take to the race track. When I questioned him further (the joys of being married to a life coach) and asked why he wanted this it came back to nostalgic memories of spending time with his Dad and uncles in the garage tinkering on cars and taking long drives in his XE Falcon to Sydney. The exact car that he wants to turn into a race car. So his big reason why was more about connection and family than just building the race car. Family is his highest value.

Step 3: Read your list daily, especially the last 10. Look at this list and see if you can find physical anchors that you can add to your everyday life. This is about becoming laser focused and using our RAS as a superpower and reminder of what it is that we want to achieve.

Just like Therese you might change the passwords on your computer or change your screensaver on the lock screen of your phone. From my examples you can see how clothes can create that connection to the emotional experiences in my life. My close friend Dr Sally Bromley had a big dream of representing Australia in dragon boating. She put the green and gold jersey on her bedroom wall as a visual reminder of her big goal. You might even use this list as the basis of your vision board.

Do you want to uplevel even further?

Take a look at the five things you do at the start of the day and the five things you do at the end of the day and see if they reflect your big reason why and goal. These are your routines and rituals. If I was to follow you around for the first part and the last part of your day I will see what you value. Does this reflect your big reason why? A fun analogy I use when working with clients is calling these your 'bookends' as bookends keep all the books together on the shelf. Just like bookends, these routines and rituals keep your life together.

Your morning bookends could look like this:

- Wake up, kiss partner and kids
- Read big reason why
- Write down goals
- Make your bed
- Train
- Take vitamins.

And your evening bookend like this:

- Pack lunch for the next day
- Read to kids in bed
- Kiss kids and partner goodnight
- Make-up off
- Write gratitude
- Meditate
- Read.

By looking at this I can see that you value your kids, your partner, health and achievement. These are your big reasons why.

Let's say that health and fitness wasn't one of your goals. You can't find the time to train because you are not scheduling it, then that shows it's not really a value. If you wanted to change this and make health and fitness a value, then you would change your morning routine.

Lucy's story

This is such a small thing. It is easy to say it's too small to matter, why should I bother? But I'd hit rock bottom and was willing to give anything a go. Here I am recovering from a car accident, evicted from a long-term home, struggling with mental health. What do I have to lose? I decided to give it a go.

The outcomes that I wanted were to work towards a cleaner house, personal growth and being healthy. I chose a few small tasks that reflected those goals. These tasks were stacked to make my morning and evening routine.

a.m.
- Make bed
- Take meds and vitamins
- Journal

p.m.
- Wash dishes, clean kitchen
- Quiet time
- Gratitude journal
- Take meds and vitamins
- Read

The difference to my mood and my wellbeing, my whole outlook on life is huge. I am now adding new things to my checklist to upgrade to the next level. This is definitely a tool I will be keeping. These small steps give you a win each day and make you want to do even more. Just like a snowball going down a mountain, it creates momentum towards your goal.

Questions from Empowered Eating clients just like you

Kim, what if I can't think of 30 reasons why?
I know that I am pushing you. This is also an exercise in commitment and to find out how bad you really want it. We are going for 30 reasons why so that you can really extend your thinking and get to your unconscious drivers. We need to get the logical brain out

of the way for a while (that's the first 20) to get to the magic. It is ok if you take a few hours or take a break and come back to it.

What if things are repeated?
This shows from your unconscious brain what is important to you. Don't ignore this special message. Ask yourself why this is important to you. Does it relate back to your childhood? Something that you missed out on or something that was meaningful to you?

Help! I don't know what goal to use?
There is no judgement here. You can't be or right or wrong, follow your heart and go with what it tells you. You can do this activity over and over for different goals. Alternately, you can keep reading and see what comes up for you from the other chapters and come back to this. Just place a post-it note here or fold the corner of the page so you don't forget.

Strategies for your Empowered Eating Toolbox

1. Have a big enough reason why so the how will take care of itself.

2. Write your 30 big reasons why you want to achieve your goal.

3. Find a way to anchor this into your everyday life. You can use physical anchors, passwords, screensavers, vision boards or anything else meaningful to you.

4. Read the last 10 reasons on your list every day.

5. Share your success with me on Facebook or Instagram.

Chapter 2

The salad is greener

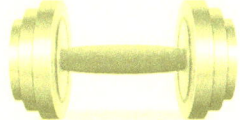

No matter who you are, no matter what you did, no matter where you've come from, you can always change, become a better version of yourself.

Madonna

One of the things I always tell myself is: I have not been put on this earth to be average. I can guarantee the exact same for you.

To stop playing average and to keep us moving in life, just like a wheel rolling down a mountain we need to continually assess where we are at. We also need to discover where we are sabotaging ourselves.

There are numerous ways that we can sabotage ourselves. In this chapter, I am going to focus on vacuums and holes in your life. When one part of our life is empty we will often unconsciously try and fill it up with unresourceful behaviour (such as binge eating).

You will notice in this book, I use the words *unresourceful behaviour* when referring to bingeing. Language is very important; it is the basis of neuro-linguistic programming. We are blaming the behaviour not the person. We are blaming your bingeing behaviour, not you. You are not a binge eater.

When you identify yourself as binger it is very hard to move from that space. When I say that you have bingeing behaviour this takes the focus away from your identity to something that is changeable. Your actions can be broken up into either resourceful or unresourceful behaviour towards your goals. We are going to focus on your resourceful behaviour and label your bingeing as unresourceful.

Now, to move you towards your goals we need to assess where you are currently sitting. Where you are playing 'average'.

To do this we are going to look at your life as if it is a wheel broken into eight areas.

During the journey of life you will find that you become absorbed in one area of life, which then creates imbalance in other areas. Being unbalanced consciously or unconsciously leads to unresourceful behaviour like bingeing.

For example, if you spend most of your time in the career area and not enough time on fun and recreation, you may emotionally eat. The reason you are emotionally eating is that you are looking for an exciting stimulus. Sugar is great for this. Momentarily you have the sugar high, you feel the rush and you feel energised.

This feeling that you are seeking, can also be created by doing something fun with friends. Just recently I started circus training as I knew I was looking for a fun high. That buzz. I could have gone back to my old behaviour of sugar highs or I could do something resourceful like doing somersaults on a trampoline for that same high.

When Kelly did this activity she had a light-bulb moment that she was seeking joy, and using food to fulfil that need. For Kelly, to fulfil that need of joy, she started going to home decor places and looking at *Home Beautiful*. This visually created joy in her life instead of looking at food to fulfil that need.

There is also the possibility of vacuums from excess in one area. Only you will know the truth. Let's look at fun and recreation in excess. By partying, going out a lot, dining and spending exorbitant money on weekends away, you may spend more time in the fun and recreation area but not enough focus on money and saving. As a result, you may find that you are not sleeping at night which makes you cranky and snappy towards your significant other or family. Having fights with your partner can lead to finding yourself in the cupboard.

When I was competing in bodybuilding, the only friends I would see were the ones that trained with me. I hardly called or saw my family, I didn't make time for fun and laughter, my career even started to slip as I was only focused on my comp prep. Next minute I was a mess: I couldn't stick to my diet, I was lacking motivation and felt alone. Eventually this all or nothing mentality shows up in your life unconsciously. By shining a torch into the dark areas we can see where your life is out of kilter and make changes for good.

Empowered Eating story time

My bodybuilding career was an interesting time in my life. My wheel was very out of balance and at times this created situations where I binged. If I looked at the wheel of life this makes a lot more sense now. I would not spend any time with my family or my friends therefore there was a vacuum in that space. When we are lacking something we fill it with something else and in my case that would be bingeing. I didn't spend time in fun and recreation because all I was doing was training to be the best body builder I could be.

My first marriage was on the rocks so therefore the area of significant other and romance had a huge vacuum as well. I'd put absolutely everything into being on stage which cost $20,000 a year in supplements, having two personal trainers, three gym memberships, hair, make-up, tanning and expensive bikinis. This created a vacuum in my financials as well.

My health was also suffering, as I was so deficient in so many vitamins and minerals. That is a whopping five areas of the wheel of life that I was out of whack, which makes sense as to why I was bingeing. I now look back and see that my wheel was very, very, clunky which meant I wasn't rolling smoothly through life. I am not against chasing big dreams or bodybuilding, just not at the detriment of every other area of your life.

Sonia's story

Sonia is a busy mum of two beautiful twin girls who is also trying to launch her hairdressing salon. When she started coaching with me she was working crazy hours to grow her business, coming home to run a household, care for her girls and be the best partner possible. She was juggling so many balls and wanting to be perfect in all of them. This is so much pressure and her soul was crying out to be nurtured and to escape the craziness of life.

Enter a bottle of wine a night. This was her way to escape. It was the only time she would sit still, unwind and chat to her husband. When we met, her goal was to look amazing in a bridesmaid's dress at her best friend's wedding. She knew that she needed to break this habit – however, because she didn't have a resourceful way to escape, she continued drinking.

When we sat down to do the wheel of life she ranked really well in the areas of environment, family, career, finances, health and growth.

She realised how much she was giving to her family and friends, her husband, her career, keeping her house tidy, going to the gym, earning and looking after the family budget and starting her journey of personal growth with me.

The one area that was missing was fun and laughter. To increase this we looked at ways in which she can make time to catch up with her friends for coffee and take some time out for herself. She sat down with her husband to schedule in me time. Me time could be spending time alone watching a funny movie, reading a book or hanging out with her friends. By simply recognising that she needed me time enabled her to show up better for her daughters, her husband and run her business effectively. By taking me time, doing something fun stopped the need to hit the bottle. They also scheduled in 10-minute power chats at the end of her day so that she could unload to the caring ear of her husband. By receiving love and connection in these power chats, it enhanced their communication, upgrading their relationship. Through these power chats they identified the need to plan date nights every fortnight and asked her sister to babysit.

Dani's story

Dani is a single parent, career woman and beautiful friend to many. She came to me because no matter how hard she tried she couldn't stick to a nutritional plan and stay on track. I wanted to find out where the vacuums were and what was stopping her from going to the next level. When we were rating all the areas of her life we discovered that her physical environment was only a 1. This was very low. I asked a few more questions about this and discovered that her house was full of clutter and her bedroom was a disaster. It resembled something of a teenage girl who was putting on a fashion show for her friends. Clothes, make-up, styling products everywhere, jumbled with her adult life of paperwork, unopened mail and that important school note for her daughter to attend school camp.

As I mentioned earlier, I have a saying that I love and use in coaching: *How do you eat an elephant? One spoonful of time.* To my clients this means they need to find the one small step they can take now to move forward. A tiny little action that will create momentum. For Dani, this meant setting a 10-minute timer to clean her room. Her one and only focus was to do just 10 minutes per day cleaning her room or other areas of her house that were cluttered. This was actionable and achievable. I wasn't asking her to clean her whole house. This also showed to her daughter that life is about repeating the little things over again and taking pride in your home space – including her bedroom and making her bed. She was finally leading by example. This became a game for them every night. Setting the timer, her daughter would go off to her room and clean and Mum would do the same.

I knew if we tackled her food she would become overwhelmed. Asking her to clean the whole house was unrealistic. She would have ended up procrastinating and not doing anything at all. By setting the tiny little task of 10 minutes per day she felt a sense of achievement and that she was making a dent in the crazy, cluttered, messy mountain.

After doing this for a few days and she reported back that not only had she cleaned up a whole room and was sleeping better, her food with back on track.

Her physical environment had a huge impact on her compliance to nutrition and not binge eating. The messy physical space made her feel overwhelmed which then created the need to soothe this feeling with food.

What are your vacuums?

Look at the areas below and rate yourself out of 10 on how you see yourself in your current situation. The middle point in the circle is 0 and the outside edge is a 10. Then join all the dots with a line forming a wonky circle. This will enable you to visually reflect and gain insight as to how you are really travelling.

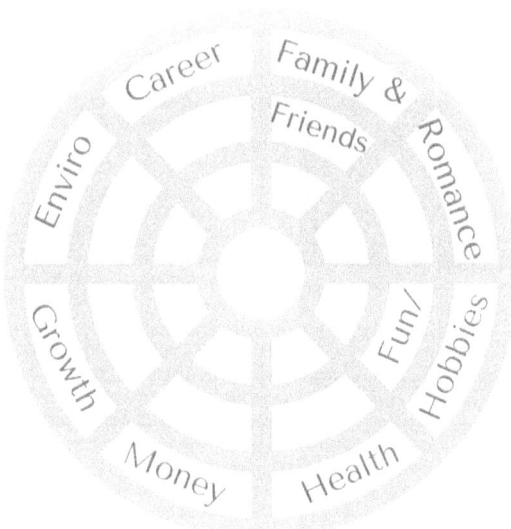

Wheel of life

It's very easy to have blinkers in life and think that we are doing great but until we actually stop and assess where we are headed, we cannot improve.

Having a balanced wheel is one of the keys to success. As you can image a wonky wheel doesn't roll very smoothly down a hill: this is you in life. To help you move at an efficient pace, we need the wheel to be balanced.

If you score an 8 to 10 in a section, congratulations! You are doing well in that area. You may have a few minor things to tweak, but overall this area of your life is complete.

If you score 5 to 7 in a section then start to put some small steps into place to bring this number up. If you score 1 to 4 in any sections then you need to ask yourself why is this so unbalanced and how is it really working for you? What steps can you take to make change before this shows up in other areas of your life?

Activity

Take some time now to write the score for each of the eight areas in the table below. If there are any areas where your score was 4 or below, write out the steps you will take to improve the balance. Let's start with three small actions per area.

Area of Life	Score
Family and friends	
Romance	
Fun and hobbies	
Health	
Money	
Growth	
Environment	
Career	

Area to improve: _____
Action 1: _____
Action 2: _____
Action 3: _____

Area to improve: _____
Action 1: _____
Action 2: _____
Action 3: _____

Area to improve: _____
Action 1: _____
Action 2: _____
Action 3: _____

Area to improve: _____
Action 1: _____
Action 2: _____
Action 3: _____

In three months' time do this exercise again and see where you score. Relate these scores back to the first wheel and against the actions you decided to take for each of the lower scores. Did you improve? Did something else fall out of balance? Who can you ask to support you to grow in this area?

Continue to reassess your direction. Life is about growing and being the best version of you.

> Life is like riding a bicycle. To keep your balance, you must keep moving.
> **Albert Einstein**

If you do the work, you will break free of your unresourceful behaviours.

(The Wheel of Life) led me to the miracle I discovered for weight loss, the end of workaholism, and to greater success than ever before.

Psychotherapist William Anderson, who lost 140 pounds after 25 years of obesity and failure with more diets than he can count.

Do you want to uplevel even further?

Success leaves clues. The areas that you scored an 8, 9 or even 10 are things you are doing really well in. This is evidence that you are capable of achieving great things. You may have hit a 9 for finances however your health was a 2 because your nutrition is out of control. We can map across from one area to the other routines and rituals that work in finance that will work with your food. An example of this might be that you budget your money but then have a little bit of play money put aside for you to spend every single week. How this evidence can be used for nutrition is that you can eat healthy 90% of the time and have that 10% for something that is not so nutritious. It might be having that glass of wine with friends.

<u>Anne's story</u>

I discussed the idea that success leaves clues in a coaching session with Anne. She had cleared 30k of debt which is no easy feat. It took dedication, commitment and hard work. She had the skill set yet she was still not being focused with her food and was falling off the bandwagon. I asked her what skills, routines and rituals she had around her money that enabled her to clear her debt so we could translate them across to her food.

The first thing we identified was her mindset. She *believed* that she could get herself out of debt, so we flicked her mindset that she can change her body composition. This is where mantras are very powerful.

She had a routine around budgeting every single week which translates to planning her meals every single week.

Daily, she tracked her abundance (things like someone buying her a coffee or not having to pay for parking) and daily expenditure like buying lunch. We translated this to keeping her food diary on MyFitnessPal.

She had money set aside each week for socialising. To mimic this, we set aside one meal a week where she socialises and it is an estimated entry in her MyFitnessPal app.

She planned upcoming events to fit in her budget. To map this across to food she looked ahead at the weddings and major social events coming up and knew that they would be the weeks that she would maintain and not expect to shift weight.

She became very comfortable with having excess money in her account and likewise it was ok to leave food on her plate. There is a correlation between those who drain their bank account and eat everything on their plate.

To find out why, check out my video on the seven links between poor money habits and poor food habits:

https://youtu.be/5q7GTmJF1_

Questions from Empowered Eating clients just like you

Kim, what if all areas are low?
Ask yourself which area would have the biggest flow on effect to other areas of your life? Would getting your finances in order and sticking to budget help catapult change? Would moving house (your environment) change everything for you? After I left my ex-husband I had a flatmate for six months. It was only when I decided that I

wanted to live on my own did my business flourish and I made the Australian Powerlifting team. This is because I had time to myself and I no longer needed to entertain a flatmate.

What if I don't know what steps to take?
Think of the easiest step to take first so this creates momentum. It could be making that phone call, booking something in, finding support, researching something. Look for the littlest tiniest step to move you forward. Movement creates momentum.

Kim! I still can't move forward.
Check out my video on Anxiety, Overwhelm and Fruit:

https://youtu.be/WbL5pp4QhCA

Strategies for your Empowered Eating Toolbox

1. If you haven't completed the activity above, take out your journal and copy the diagram. Don't forget to add the date. I have a few wheels that don't have dates and now I am kicking myself. Rate each area.

2. Look at your wheel and write down any areas that are below a 4. You need to address this immediately.

3. For every area that is below a 4, you need to uncover three steps to move you forward.

Chapter 3

What really matters?

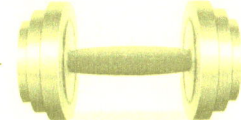

> Happiness in life is achieved through two things: growth as a human being and living according to our values.
>
> Unknown

Not living according to your values causes mental, emotional and physical suffering. It can lead to sleepless nights, headaches, anxiety and a long list of ailments – which can then lead to emotional eating.

I experienced this firsthand myself. I had a fantastic salary position as the PT manager for a well-known gym chain. Those that have worked in the fitness industry, know that salary jobs are few and far between. To receive holiday pay, sick pay and a regular income each week is an absolute dream. However, after working in this job for nine months, I was constantly feeling exhausted, irritable and sick. I would wake up in the morning and it would be such a struggle to get out of bed even though I was doing the job that I absolutely loved. Being a personal trainer was my heart and soul.

I had a deep conversation with myself in my journal. This is the reason why I encourage you to journal as you will find your own answers. I asked myself what was really going on here. Why was I always sick and why was I exhausted doing what I loved? Something was incongruent.

That word *incongruent* set alarm bells off! Remember the opening quote at the start of this chapter? *Happiness in life is achieved through two things: growth as a human being and living according to our values.* I had learnt this in my life coaching certification and I knew its power. So much so that I had etched it permanently in my brain.

The incongruence was in the way I was receiving my income. The company I was working for, valued money over clients. All they cared about was how much money I could make them as a personal trainer. To meet the hefty targets they had set as my KPIs as a condition of my salary meant I was clocking in 50 sessions a week while managing staff. Emotionally I was spread really thin. I was losing the authenticity and connection that was my unique point of difference. My clients deserve my full attention and emotional space to feel valued – not feeling like a number being pushed through the queue like a conveyor belt in a factory.

The reason I started this career in 2006 was to change people's lives. I couldn't do that when I was tired, exhausted and worried about making enough money to make my boss happy. Making an impact on people's lives is my highest value and hence why you are reading this book. Once I had this light-bulb moment I quit my very sought-after salary job to start my own business. I instantly felt energised and started to love life again. That's when I knew I had made the right decision to live according to my values.

Not being clear on your values is very dangerous. You can easily fall into a spiral of taking on other people's values and what they think of you, not standing in your space and living an authentic life. A life according to your values. Personal values are the things that are important to us, the characteristics and behaviours that motivate us and guide our decisions. When you become clear on what your values are, then decision-making is easy. Just like my decision to quit.

In some situations you may be able to make short-term changes, but if it violates your values then you will become unhappy. For example, you may wish to compete in an iron man – but if you value family and training takes up too much family time, then you may become unhappy and unmotivated through the process. Training will become a struggle.

Vivian's story

Living congruently with your values will open more pathways for success. Vivian messaged me after an episode of bingeing because she had not been successful in her promotion at work. I was able to offer her an emergency appointment and we unpacked what was really going on. I had an inkling that she hadn't given her all in the job application and the interview. When I asked about her prep for the interview she admitted that she hadn't spent as long as she had wanted on her resume because her daughter was playing in the basketball grand final. She went and watched the game, leaving writing her resume to the last minute.

I asked her a little bit more about the position that she had applied for, it required her going from part-time to full-time.

This meant that she couldn't pick her kids up from school and would miss out on that valuable chat that comes organically over afternoon tea and helping them with their homework. For her, being there for her children was about being a mother who is present. The exact opposite to what she grew up with – an alcoholic father and a working mother.

I asked her to pull out her values worksheet and tell me what her top five values were. Family was her number one value as I had expected. We were able to alleviate some of the pain from missing out on the promotion because it wasn't congruent with her number one value which is being a 100% present mother for her children.

She just so happened to be talking to another mother the following week about understanding her values and missing out on the promotion. This mother told her about a position at a not-for-profit organisation that was part-time and the offering salary was much higher than what Vivian was receiving. Now she is working for an organisation that aligns with her values, while giving back to the community. And she can still do school pickups.

Your values are the key

You never know what doors will open up when you start living according to your values. Like when I became clear on the message that I wanted to make women emotionally, mentally and physically strong. Being strong is one of my values, and when married with my value of helping people, more podcasts, radio interviews and media opportunities came my way. It is also the reason why you have this book in your hot little hands.

Becoming clear on what you value means you won't second guess your choices in life and you will start to back yourself more. When

I met my biological father for the first time and discovered that he is a drug addict, I didn't second guess my decision to cut him out of my life. I was able to stand in my space and know that I didn't want that in my life. He violated many of my other core and religious values as well, making this choice logical in an emotional time. From this, you can understand how knowing your values will simplify decision-making on matters of great importance. That feeling of being unsettled over decisions will also ease when you know your highest values.

A few questions to help you define what you value

What do you get on your soapbox about?
I value loyalty and trust so when people lie and cheat it makes me very angry. This is also a reflection of the pain caused by some early ex-boyfriends who shattered my self-esteem by cheating.

What do you spend your time and money on?
I value my career and won't think twice about spending $5000 on a training course. Education and knowledge means I can help others.

What things do you talk about/ bang on and on about? What is it about this that you value?
I will talk about training and personal development until the cows come home. I value health, fitness and self-development.

What results do you get in your life? What would others say your life produces?
I value achievement, so I won't let anything get in the way of training for Worlds, it is the first priority over socialising, work, everything except my husband, and thankfully he understands my highest values. I would suggest that you also talk to your significant other about your values. This will help prevent future arguments. My husband is Greek and I knew before marrying him that family is his highest value. We never have any arguments over family as I love

and respect his highest value. It goes both ways, he knows that lifting will always be a part of my life which means that some of our overseas holidays will be to locations that I am competing at. Four months after our wedding we were in Japan so I could compete at Worlds. We forfeited having a honeymoon immediately after the wedding because prepping for Worlds was my highest value.

Activity

Grab a pen and go through this list and circle the values that resonates with you.

1. Abundance
2. Acceptance
3. Accessibility
4. Accomplishment
5. Accountability
6. Accuracy
7. Achievement
8. Acknowledgement
9. Activeness
10. Adaptability
11. Adoration
12. Adroitness
13. Advancement
14. Adventure
15. Affection
16. Affluence
17. Aggressiveness
18. Agility
19. Alertness
20. Altruism
21. Amazement
22. Ambition
23. Amusement
24. Anticipation
25. Appreciation
26. Approachability
27. Approval
28. Art
29. Articulacy
30. Artistry
31. Assertiveness
32. Assurance
33. Attentiveness
34. Attractiveness
35. Audacity
36. Availability
37. Awareness
38. Awe
39. Balance
40. Beauty
41. Being the best
42. Belonging
43. Benevolence
44. Bliss
45. Boldness
46. Bravery
47. Brilliance
48. Buoyancy
49. Calmness
50. Camaraderie
51. Candour
52. Capability
53. Care
54. Carefulness
55. Celebrity
56. Certainty
57. Challenge
58. Change
59. Charity
60. Charm
61. Chastity
62. Cheerfulness
63. Clarity
64. Cleanliness
65. Clear-mindedness
66. Cleverness

67. Closeness
68. Comfort
69. Commitment
70. Community
71. Compassion
72. Competence
73. Competition
74. Completion
75. Composure
76. Concentration
77. Confidence
78. Conformity
79. Congruency
80. Connection
81. Consciousness
82. Conservation
83. Consistency
84. Contentment
85. Continuity
86. Contribution
87. Control
88. Conviction
89. Conviviality
90. Coolness
91. Cooperation
92. Cordiality
93. Correctness
94. Country
95. Courage
96. Courtesy
97. Craftiness
98. Creativity
99. Credibility
100. Cunning
101. Curiosity
102. Daring

103. Decisiveness
104. Decorum
105. Deference
106. Delight
107. Dependability
108. Depth
109. Desire
110. Determination
111. Devotion
112. Devoutness
113. Dexterity
114. Dignity
115. Diligence
116. Direction
117. Directness
118. Discipline
119. Discovery
120. Discretion
121. Diversity
122. Dominance
123. Dreaming
124. Drive
125. Duty
126. Dynamism
127. Eagerness
128. Ease
129. Economy
130. Ecstasy
131. Education
132. Effectiveness
133. Efficiency
134. Elation
135. Elegance
136. Empathy
137. Encouragement
138. Endurance

139. Energy
140. Enjoyment
141. Entertainment
142. Enthusiasm
143. Environmentalism
144. Ethics
145. Euphoria
146. Excellence
147. Excitement
148. Exhilaration
149. Expectancy
150. Expediency
151. Experience
152. Expertise
153. Exploration
154. Expressiveness
155. Extravagance
156. Extroversion
157. Exuberance
158. Fairness
159. Faith
160. Fame
161. Family
162. Fascination
163. Fashion
164. Fearlessness
165. Ferocity
166. Fidelity
167. Fierceness
168. Financial independence
169. Firmness
170. Fitness
171. Flexibility
172. Flow
173. Fluency

174. Focus
175. Fortitude
176. Frankness
177. Freedom
178. Friendliness
179. Friendship
180. Frugality
181. Fun
182. Gallantry
183. Generosity
184. Gentility
185. Giving
186. Grace
187. Gratitude
188. Gregariousness
189. Growth
190. Guidance
191. Happiness
192. Harmony
193. Health
194. Heart
195. Helpfulness
196. Heroism
197. Holiness
198. Honesty
199. Honour
200. Hopefulness
201. Hospitality
202. Humility
203. Humour
204. Hygiene
205. Imagination
206. Impact
207. Impartiality
208. Independence
209. Individuality
210. Industry
211. Influence
212. Ingenuity
213. Inquisitiveness
214. Insightfulness
215. Inspiration
216. Integrity
217. Intellect
218. Intelligence
219. Intensity
220. Intimacy
221. Intrepidness
222. Introspection
223. Introversion
224. Intuition
225. Intuitiveness
226. Inventiveness
227. Investing
228. Involvement
229. Joy
230. Judiciousness
231. Justice
232. Keenness
233. Kindness
234. Knowledge
235. Leadership
236. Learning
237. Liberation
238. Liberty
239. Lightness
240. Liveliness
241. Logic
242. Longevity
243. Love
244. Loyalty
245. Majesty
246. Making a difference
247. Marriage
248. Mastery
249. Maturity
250. Meaning
251. Meekness
252. Mellowness
253. Meticulousness
254. Mindfulness
255. Modesty
256. Motivation
257. Mysteriousness
258. Nature
259. Neatness
260. Nerve
261. Nonconformity
262. Obedience
263. Open-mindedness
264. Openness
265. Optimism
266. Order
267. Organisation
268. Originality
269. Outdoors
270. Outlandishness
271. Outrageousness
272. Partnership
273. Patience
274. Passion
275. Peace
276. Perceptiveness
277. Perfection
278. Perkiness
279. Perseverance
280. Persistence

281. Persuasiveness
282. Philanthropy
283. Piety
284. Playfulness
285. Pleasantness
286. Pleasure
287. Poise
288. Polish
289. Popularity
290. Potency
291. Power
292. Practicality
293. Pragmatism
294. Precision
295. Preparedness
296. Presence
297. Pride
298. Privacy
299. Proactivity
300. Professionalism
301. Prosperity
302. Prudence
303. Punctuality
304. Purity
305. Rationality
306. Realism
307. Reason
308. Reasonableness
309. Recognition
310. Recreation
311. Refinement
312. Reflection
313. Relaxation
314. Reliability
315. Relief
316. Religiousness
317. Reputation
318. Resilience
319. Resolution
320. Resolve
321. Resourcefulness
322. Respect
323. Responsibility
324. Rest
325. Restraint
326. Reverence
327. Richness
328. Rigor
329. Sacredness
330. Sacrifice
331. Sagacity
332. Saintliness
333. Sanguinity
334. Satisfaction
335. Science
336. Security
337. Self-control
338. Selflessness
339. Self-reliance
340. Self-respect
341. Sensitivity
342. Sensuality
343. Serenity
344. Service
345. Sexiness
346. Sexuality
347. Sharing
348. Shrewdness
349. Significance
350. Silence
351. Silliness
352. Simplicity
353. Sincerity
354. Skilfulness
355. Solidarity
356. Solitude
357. Sophistication
358. Soundness
359. Speed
360. Spirit
361. Spirituality
362. Spontaneity
363. Spunk
364. Stability
365. Status
366. Stealth
367. Stillness
368. Strength
369. Structure
370. Success
371. Support
372. Supremacy
373. Surprise
374. Sympathy
375. Synergy
376. Teaching
377. Teamwork
378. Temperance
379. Thankfulness
380. Thoroughness
381. Thoughtfulness
382. Thrift
383. Tidiness
384. Timeliness
385. Traditionalism
386. Tranquillity
387. Transcendence
388. Trust

389. Trustworthiness
390. Truth

From there, list your top 10 below:

1) _____

2) _____

3) _____

4) _____

5) _____

6) _____

7) _____

8) _____

9) _____

10) _____

Identifying your true values can be difficult, but be honest and look deep inside yourself. This is a really important step, because knowing which value is more important is a powerful guide in times when you are faced with a decision where the options may satisfy two or more of your different values.

Look at your top two values and ask yourself, 'If I could satisfy only one of these, which would I choose?'. It might help to visualise a situation in which you would have to make that choice. For example you may have been offered two events management jobs. Job A is at a corporate organisation with a high salary and Job B is at a charity organisation for a lower salary. If you're comparing values of financial security versus impact on the world, which is more important to you?

Once you've identified your top-priority values, check that they fit with your life and your vision for yourself. Do they make you feel good about yourself? Do you feel a sense of pride about your top three values? Would you be comfortable to share them with your family, friends and others that you respect and admire? Do your values accurately represent things you would support, even if it means you are in the minority?

By considering your values when making decisions, you can keep your integrity intact and do what is right. You'll approach decision-making with clarity and feel confident that what you're doing is best for you now and in the future.

Making value-based choices can be hard at the time – but it pays off in the long run, knowing you have made the right choice.

Do you want to uplevel even further?

After prioritising your values take out your journal and write about the following:

1. What came up for you during this process?
2. What experiences do you have where your values were violated? Forgive and release these. Writing forgiveness letters will help.
3. What changes will you make?
4. Do you need to discuss this new knowledge with family, your significant other and boss?
5. What examples do you have where you lived according to your values?

Questions from Empowered Eating clients just like you

Kim I feel like my values are the same as my parents and I am recreating their values. Is this normal?
The way we were raised greatly influences our values in the present. It is up to you as an adult to decide if that value still serves you.

I am struggling to identify my values, what should I do?
When going through the list above circle the ones that first jump out at you then follow up with questions like why is that important to me? What is so special about that? Who do I want to be remembered as?

My values aren't the same as my partner's. What should I do?
Sorry to burst your bubble but you are not the same as your partner. You are 100% unique because of your life experience, you came from a different map of the world, you were raised in a different family and you have different memories. All these factors shape your values.

Strategies for your Empowered Eating Toolbox

1. When you are next faced with a big decision, go back to your values and ask yourself are you being congruent with your values.

2. Review your weekend. Are you being congruent with your values with how you use your time and money?

3. If you feel like bingeing, ask yourself, 'Am I living congruently with my values? Are any of my values being violated?'. This is your secret key to understanding some of the unconscious reasons why you sabotage your results.

Chapter 4

Owning you

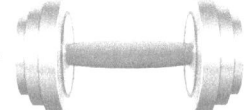

> Beneath the surface-level fears around failure, disappointment and rejection, lies our deepest fear. The fear of not being enough. This fear is often far harder to see, but part of overcoming all insecurity is about turning the lights on so you can see exactly what you are fighting.
>
> Jaemin Frazer

Every time you face your fears, you will increase your self-esteem. I have moved interstate (including living at Uluru) four times in my adult life and every single time I was facing the fear of making new friends, not knowing the area, getting lost, being isolated from family and the overriding fear of *what if I fail*. I definitely feel that pushing through this has contributed to my high levels of self-esteem and confidence.

For those who love brain science, research shows 'a preferential response of the dopaminergic midbrain to stimulus novelty'. This may indicate 'a special biological relevance for novelty as motivating' (Kakade and Dayan, 2002, Schultz, 1998).

Novelty can be interpreted as fear or something that you do not know.

We all have fears; it's part of human nature as it keeps us safe. It keeps us comfortable. However, sometimes, it stops us from living life at a higher level. I'm not talking about the fear of going into a dark alley by ourselves in the middle of the night – this fear has a purpose, as it keeps us from being mugged and hurt. I'm talking about the fears in our unconscious that we continue to accept and follow even though there doesn't seem to be any real gain from it. Some coaches like to call these secondary gains. These are fears we hold onto and it creates a behaviour that produces an undesirable outcome. We don't know why we hold onto this fear, but doing so outweighs the perceived gain. As humans we don't do anything unless there is a reward for it, and we don't do things unless it works for us (secondary gain).

> The reality is, we are exactly where we have chosen to be. Every negative thing in our life we don't like, but haven't removed, must be working for us on some level. It creates a certainty of feeling and a way of behaving.
> ***Jaemin Frazer***

Most fears come back to one of the following:

- Feeling like a fraud
- Fear of success
- Fear of failure
- Fear of being unsafe
- Fear of responsibility

- Fear of rejection
- Fear of loss of love
- Fear of loss of income
- Fear of judgement
- Fear of missing out
- Needing to look good
- Needing to be right
- Needing to feel significant
- Needing to be comfortable.

Take emotional eating for example. This comes up a lot in coaching as the number one habit that's holding someone back from achieving their goals, to the point of self-sabotaging. What if you let go of emotional eating? Who would you need to be? Sometimes when we unpack the habit, it comes down to a fear of success or a need to feel comfortable. If you were in the best possible shape of your life you may get a little more attention than usual. This attention may make you feel uncomfortable. So, you continue to binge eat as it makes you feel comfortable and no longer visible.

Think of this body fat as protection. It is protecting you from something. To set yourself free you must discover what it is that you are protecting yourself from.

Empowered Eating story time

I have two extreme examples of this from coaching. The first example is of Linda who was sexually abused as a child and she was using her marshmallow suit as a protective layer. This protective layer is body fat which she thought made her unattractive to the opposite sex. Because of the abuse she needed to be as unattractive as possible so that no-one could hurt her again.

Until she felt comfortable standing in her space and being able to protect herself there was no way that she was ever going to change her body composition. As her coach, I knew I needed to give her as many tools as possible to help her move forward.

We did two exercises in my Empowered Eating Masterclass where I bought in a professional kickboxer to teach the real basics of self-defence. This lesson included five basic moves to escape a perpetrator. We practised these moves over and over, to know how as women, we can safely get out of a hold or a sticky situation. The one that stuck in Linda's mind was where a perpetrator is lying on top of her and doing 'The Prawn'. This is how to prawn our way out of this particular hold – where you move your hips up and out from under them. Think shifting your bottom as far back as possible away from them while turning your hip and kicking the hell out of them. Google BJJ or self-defence shrimp move (I'm Australian, we call it a prawn) to gain a full understanding of this effective technique, so you too can have confidence.

The next activity I organised with the group was for us all to walk up and make sleazy comments as if we were trying to pick her up in a bar. I told Linda to square off her shoulders, stand upright with strong posture. Posture is everything as your physiology will depict how your voice sounds. It also means that you take up more physical space. Have you ever seen an alpha male in action around his friends? He stands tall and wide, squaring his shoulders. By changing her physiology, she spoke completely differently. She also practised saying no in a firm voice. This was the first time Linda had ever stood in her own space and pushed back against those that made her feel uncomfortable. My sole purpose of these two sessions was to make her feel safe in standing in her space and setting boundaries. These tools were necessary for her confidence and long-term success in shifting weight.

If this story is familiar to you please seek help from a psychologist to deal with the trauma. I would also encourage you to learn self-defence. The unconscious reason I was drawn to powerlifting and bodybuilding was that it made me feel safe that I could finally protect myself. I was physically strong and couldn't easily be pushed around. Something I couldn't do as a child, living in domestic violence. If you ever get to meet me in person you will see that I have strong upright posture and take up space because of how muscular I am.

There is also further research to back up the association between posture and confidence. The more upright you are the more serotonin you have pumping around your body. Serotonin is our feel-good hormone.

The more I can encourage you to know how to protect yourself and to stand in your space, the closer you are to shedding your protective marshmallow suit.

The second example comes from a client who had a massive fear of being visible and standing out for different reasons. She feared that if she became attractive and received a lot of attention from the opposite sex she would cheat on her husband. By making herself unattractive she wasn't receiving compliments and attention from the opposite sex, which meant the temptation to cheat on her husband was less.

Both these ladies have a fear of being visible. Being visible isn't safe and caused great emotional harm. Until you find the unconscious driver as to why you are sabotaging your results it will be challenging to stop your binge eating behaviour.

I learnt the hard way. When your body is in such a high-stress, high-cortisol state, you cannot change your body composition as the only fuel source that your body will utilise is carbohydrates. Carbs are the fuel for fight or flight response and when there is no carbs left then it will use muscle stores that you worked so hard for, which also decreases your metabolism as muscle burns calories. When you are stressed, highly strung or anxious it will not touch your fat stores, only carbs. Stress keeps you fat.

What about the fear of success?

Living life at a higher level is very daunting. You need to take responsibility for your actions; people may have greater expectations of you. For Kaitlin this meant playing it small in her public service job and not chasing the next promotion. Because if she earnt a higher wage, she would be expected to move out of home and become fully responsible for her own life, including her failures.

As human beings we have two driving forces: to Look Good and Be Right (thank you to Landmark Education for that great quote). This creates a habit of playing small and not trying. *What if you fail!* Failing would make you look bad. We must always look good. So, it's much easier to not try.

The reality is we are exactly where we have chosen to be. Every negative thing in our life we don't like, but haven't removed must be working for us on some level. It creates a certainty of feeling and a way of behaving. Identify the positive intent.

Being an unhealthy size that reduces your physical capability can be used as manipulation. For Tamara, she could barely bathe her son, put clothes on the line, sweep the house or make the bed without being out of breath. Her partner did everything around the house, because Tamara had limited movement and become tired easily. She also controlled the social situations. She didn't attend certain events as she was embarrassed about her size, this included an awards night for her husband because she didn't want to be seen by his work friends. Tamara's family feels sorry for her because she saw things she shouldn't have as a kid and is now hiding away from the world. She gets to manipulate the world around her and it works. In our coaching session she took full responsibility for manipulating those around her, apologised to her husband and day by day is changing her actions. Without identifying this secondary gain we would never have leveraged change.

Procrastination is another challenge that comes up in coaching. By not attending to the things around the house on that to-do list could mean that you need to forgo a few social gatherings which may mean that they don't need to see the extra kilos you have gained from emotional eating. You are essentially checking out of life, which works as you won't be judged.

You could also be using procrastination as a 'screw you' to your parents. By procrastinating, your parents don't get to take credit for your success. This was true for Talia. Growing up her mother wasn't present in the rearing of her own children, she didn't participate in raising the kids as the bottle was more important. Publicly, she would brag about them yet at home she was nasty, telling them that they were good for nothing, would never amount to anything in their lives and a whole host of other horrible destructive programming. This verbal abuse was part of everyday life for Talia. When Talia succeeded at becoming school captain in year 12 her mother bragged to her friends at the pub, taking credit for raising such a strong daughter. Her daughter was only strong because of all the pain she endured. Overhearing this infuriated Talia. At this age she had become very aware of how little parenting her mother had done. Right then and there she decided she would take the ball from her mother's court and never do anything that her mother could claim to be a result of her great parenting skills or could paint herself as the saintly mother. In Talia's words, 'How dare you take credit for something you didn't create? Screw you'. This was a form of control. By procrastinating she was able to control her mother.

Another example is going for that dream job. What if you get rejected? What if you fail the interview? This would make you look bad. Rejection feels like the first time when you didn't get the job at Sportsgirl as a teenager. You cried all day and the popular girl at school who worked there, knew you went for the job and made fun of you on Monday.

What if you lose your current income? I had this fear when I left my salary job to start my online business working for myself. There was a great fear around safety and security. What if I didn't make it? What if I failed? If I failed it would look bad going back and asking my employer for my position again. I wanted to stay comfortable, stay average. Being safe is the secondary gain.

By addressing the secondary gain, we are able to see the light, and then change our behaviours. We have the freedom to choose a new behaviour that meets the positive intent in better ways.

Activity

Time to grab a pen and answer the following questions in the space below or in your journal:

What is the one thing that is holding you back from achieving your best life?

___

What are the payoffs?

___

What is the good thing about this?

___

What do you get from avoiding dealing with this?

___

What is stopping you from making that change?

_____

What is the fear behind this?

_____

Is this fear real? Or false evidence appearing real?

_____

What are some logical reasons to change?

_____

What would your life look like if you eliminated this fear?

_____

Who do you need to be to live the life that you imagined?

_____

What three steps could you take to start living that life?

_____

As philosopher William James observed, *most people live in a restricted circle of potential.*

Playing small means you miss out on the honey of life, the little extra that other people enjoy. Face your fears and you too, can taste the honey.

Do you want to uplevel even further?

Look back into your childhood and see where these fears come from. Look for three examples for each fear. Journal first through your child (mini me) eyes and then through the eyes of an adult and see if the adult can pass on any knowledge or gifts of how to meet mini me's needs. Did mini me need love, support, encouragement, safety? How can you provide that for them now, as you the adult?

Questions from Empowered Eating clients just like you

Kim, what if I can't figure out my fear?
Look at the list of fears and journal about one that jumps out at you. Ask your soul, what is it keeping you safe from? Still can't find your fears? Look at a family member or your best friend. Think of a behaviour that they are doing that keeps them safe. Then look at your own life and see if you have a story that relates

What if my fears are from traumatic events?
You may need professional help from a trained psychologist and this is ok. Talk to them about this book and what came up for you. There is nothing to be ashamed of. Most successful people I know have seen a psychologist at one point in their life. I was in therapy for three years to deal with mine. Why spend your whole life battling this when they could fix it in a few sessions?

Strategies for your Empowered Eating Toolbox

1. Spend time journaling.

2. Answer the questions with as much detail as possible. The deeper you go, the better the transformation and the more you will learn about yourself.

3. Thank your fears for keeping you safe.

4. Look for little ways that you can face your fears. This could be talking to the person in line at the petrol station.

5. List all the resources and steps you can take to tackle your fears.

Chapter 5

Sexy and confident

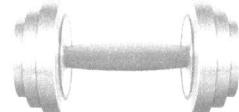

You idiot, you're such a failure, no wonder you are so fat. Look at the cellulite! Why can't you just stay in control, you useless piece of crap.

The above dialogue is tame compared to some of the things that we say to ourselves. I know because I did it and I know you do too. This self-talk is so disgusting we wouldn't even talk to our pet fish like that!

This must change. Those nasty words are the real reason you can't stop bingeing. How we speak to ourselves directly impacts what our unconscious mind believes. When you are saying horrible comments to yourself your unconscious mind believes exactly what you are telling it. Every muscle in your body believes it, every cell feels it, and this then changes your physiology. The change in physiology changes your actions and habits, which ultimately becomes your reality.

As Gandhi said:

Your beliefs become your thoughts,
Your thoughts become your words,
Your words become your actions,
Your actions become your habits,
Your habits become your values,
Your values become your destiny.

What I want for you is for you to become your own best friend. I want you to start to believe that you are beautiful, sexy and confident – and it starts with how you talk to yourself.

Because you have spoken so harshly to yourself for so long we need to take drastic action to change your language. Language is the basics of neuro-linguistic programming (NLP). Like a computer program, you are being coded by your language. Let's create effective coding that changes you from an unconscious level. We are going to create mantras that you can say to yourself every day.

Where attention goes, energy flows and results follow. By repeating your mantras daily, you are helping unlock subconscious beliefs which lead to unresourceful behaviours like bingeing. Repeating a positive statement to yourself reinforces positive actions. Repetition is the mother of all skills, so you are going to repeat your mantra numerous times a day. Trust me this works. To be world-class at benching I must do 1000s of reps in the gym.

Find your mantra

My favourite statement that I use to this day is: 'I deserve success'. We are going to create an environmental trigger by identifying where you are going to say this mantra. You could repeat your statement when you are driving to work, brushing your teeth, walking the dog or any other daily mindless activity.

One of my beautiful clients writes her mantra on the steam that forms on the shower screen in her bathroom! Best idea ever! One of my old behaviours was to self-sabotage. The moment things were going well I would do something to sabotage my result. I needed to reprogram my subconscious mind. It took practice, but my mantra, *I deserve success* is repeated to this day. I can now feel when I am going to slip up and I sternly repeat my mantra. Some others that my clients have used include:

- I am enough
- I love and approve of myself
- I am worthy
- It's safe for me to be successful
- It's safe to be visible
- I get sh@# done
- Just do it.

Which phrase resonates with you and can help rewrite that negative story that you tell yourself? Write it down and turn it into your mantra – it should always be positive words. Try and say it at least 10 times a day. There may be specific times that you say it like when you brush your teeth, when you write in your gratitude journal, on particular parts of your drive to work, when you feel like you are on the verge of sabotaging or before you eat every meal. Just like a computer we are going to reprogram your unconscious mind and install a better update. If Microsoft Windows can have updates and new versions, so can you.

A fun way to work with this is to name your nasty side, turning it into a character. You can talk to this character and tell it to shut up. This also works for anxiety or the little voice that wants to binge. You can ask them to leave. By naming this behaviour it takes out the emotion and changes thought patterns. A client of mine calls hers 'the witch from Snow White', another calls her 'DQ' which stands for drama queen. An extreme version is my client who sees his inner voice as a ringmaster that whips him when he talks nasty to himself. He backs this up with a flick of a rubber band that is permanently on his wrist. If you are like me and get pulled towards pleasure you can use a fun alter ego. A few of my clients have alter egos of Crystalina the Great, Hot Mumma and Warrior Zelda. Who is your alter ego? What is the identity of the person who you want to be?

In the words of well-known change coach Tony Robbins:

> *Incantations are powerful! You can't just get rid of a negative belief; you have to replace it. Try incanting your new beliefs, saying them again and again, changing the emphasis and changing your state. By changing the emotion, you change the impact you feel and you begin to condition yourself for even more action.*

To be binge-free, we must become familiar with the new belief, the new mantra — because when the mind is left to its own devices, it rejects the unfamiliar and returns to the familiar because it is safe. By repeating your mantras you are becoming familiar and comfortable with the new way of believing and being.

An important part of our journey together is that I want you to believe that *you are worthy, that you love yourself and you are enough*. Mantras, or as Tony Robbins calls them, incantations, are where we start, then we take it next level and supercharge it. To do this we are going to look at ways to make these neurological pathways even stronger by taking actions towards self-love in a way that your brain understands.

The language of love

Let me introduce you to my favourite book in the whole world, *The 5 Love Languages* by marriage counsellor Gary Chapman.

In this amazing book Gary talks about the five different ways different people express love.

They are:

- **Words or affirmations.** Building someone up with sincere compliments.
- **Spending time.** Spending quality time with someone and giving them our undivided attention.
- **Giving and receiving gifts.** A gift is something that you can hold in your hand and say this person was thinking of me. It doesn't need to cost money, a flower from the garden shows that you were thinking of them.
- **Acts of service.** Doing things for another person or helping them with something.
- **Physical touch.** Hugs, kisses, hand on the shoulder, holding hands, even play fighting.

It's important to first know your own. Some individuals will instantly know their own love language, but for others it will not be that easy.

If you need some help working it out, think about these questions:

What makes you feel loved?

What do you desire above all else?

How do you express love to others?

What do people do or not do that hurts you deeply?

Considering these questions and thinking about your answers should help you work out what your love language is. Chances are, how you show your love to others is also your own love language.

If you would like a more accurate result take the test: https://www.5lovelanguages.com/profile/singles/

I often refer to the five love languages in coaching sessions and clients have taken this information and used it to help improve relationships in all areas of their life, reducing the need to soothe broken relationships with food.

Self-love is showing you that you love you. We are going to talk to your brain in the language that it understands. Binge eating isn't self-love, it's more like an abusive relationship. We don't do that anymore. Abuse may be something you endured as a child, but as an adult you are not going to keep this pattern going. You are going to become familiar with what love feels like, how to show up for yourself and love yourself from the core with the help of Gary's book.

If acts of service are important to you then those little things all add up. Show you that you love and respect yourself by making the bed every morning. You may organise for someone to wash your car or have a housekeeper. Learn how to apply make-up for a new look. Light candles at night. By doing the little things you are showing you that you matter.

Maybe your love language is gifts. You love buying other people gifts so why aren't you buying yourself gifts? A nice bottle of perfume, some new lingerie, a new recipe book, a candle or pick flowers from the garden. These things don't need to be expensive; they are physical anchors that you will see daily reminding yourself that you love you.

If positive affirmations are important to you, start with listening to your own self-talk. How positive is it? Is it the way you would talk to someone that you love or are you treating yourself like dirt? The whole section at the start of this chapter would have really hit you hard in the heart if this is your love language. Some positive mantras that I use regularly are, 'I deserve love and success', 'I'm happy and sparkly' and 'I love my own unique self'.

Spending time is my prominent language so I will take myself on self-dates. I'll go to the movies alone because I deserve that. I'll treat myself to a good meal out or take my dog for a walk up the mountain. Go to a Bikram class, drive to Coogee or simply lay on the grass and daydream. It's this free time to think and spend time alone, because my time matters.

My secondary love language is physical touch (usually you have a primary and secondary). I love hugs, to be held and have my hair played with. By knowing this I show myself how much I love myself by making a body scrub of coffee and salt then slathering myself in coconut oil, I wear good quality clothes that feel good on my skin and love lying on the sand or grass in the sun, feeling the warmth on my back. This is also spending time with myself and being in the present.

When you discover which love languages speak to you and put it into practice it improves your own self-confidence straight away.

Find time for you

When it comes to making time for self-love, I often hear the excuse that, 'I don't have time for me' or sometimes my clients who have children feel guilty for taking time out. In reality, if you are a mum and you are saying that your family is suffering because you're not in your best state, you owe it to them and to you to *make the time*. It's likely Mum is hard to deal with when she is frazzled and tired.

You know when you are on a plane and they tell you, 'in an emergency, always fit your own oxygen mask before helping the person next to you' – well it applies in life too. At the stage you are in right now you have nothing left to give. You cannot give from empty. A cranky, snappy, unhappy, person who soothes with food. By nurturing your soul, you become a better partner, boss and mother. By filling up your cup, you will increase your productivity and earning capacity because you are in flow.

Love does not erase the past but it makes the future different. When we choose to actively express the primary love language to ourselves then we show us that we are important in our life. We can grow in confidence and love within ourselves and also in our love for others.

Activity

Ways to nurture your soul. Take 10 minutes to yourself right now and write a list of 30 things that nurture your soul and align with your love languages. You will probably find that you have two prominent love languages but, I would also suggest brainstorming a few more so that you cover all five.

1) _____

2) _____

3) _____

4) _____

5) _____

6) _____

7) _____

8) _____

9) _____

10) _____

11) _____

12) _____

13) _____

14) _____

15) _____

16) _____

17) _____

18) _____

19) _____

20) _____

21) _____

22) _____

23) _____

24) _____

25) _____

26) _____

27) _____

28) _____

29) _____

30) _____

Self-care plus self-awareness equals self-love. When you love and nurture yourself you don't soothe with food.

Self-care existed long before millennials did. Ancient Greeks saw it as a way to make people more honest citizens who were more likely to care for others.

Empowered Eating story time

Having not grown up with a biological father or a significant role model in my life I didn't feel loved. It took me until I was 30 something to realise that the only person that could love me is me. Yes I had a crap childhood and didn't feel loved but I couldn't continue to blame other people for my inadequacies.

Being unfamiliar to feeling loved and enough, it had to come from me. I stopped outsourcing my need for approval and love from other people and started to look at all the different ways that I could love myself. *The 5 Love Languages* really opened my mind as to what was possible and all the different ways that I could show me that I love me. I know I am enough because I love me and no-one can take that away from me.

I do absolutely believe in the cliché that until you love yourself, you cannot find a partner to love you. I spent my early thirties really working on my self-worth and ability to like and love myself. I started with like and then moved to love. If I hadn't done this serious groundwork then I would not be married to my wonderful husband as I would have found another guy that I needed to rescue or who would treat me bad. I believe within my soul I am worthy of love and that I can provide that infinite love. If the source comes from within then that is what makes me attractive to my partner.

I also looked at my origin story as to why I didn't feel lovable. When was the first time I learnt that I was unlovable? Major coding happens between the ages of 0 to 7. This is where you will find your first origin story. For me my origin story is my biological father left when I was two and it made me believe that I wasn't worthy and I didn't deserve love, success or happiness. This is my core thought and belief about myself that has come about from a two-year-old who doesn't understand why my father left and has abandoned me. From there I believed that I wasn't worthy and I wasn't good enough. My whole life was based on the experiences and beliefs of a two-year-old. I then spent the rest of my life finding more and more evidence that I was unlovable.

Fast forward to where I was in school and I broke my sandals. I came from Queensland, sandals are summer shoes. My mum was really, really angry at me, at the time I didn't know her anger was from not knowing how she was going to afford to replace them. From Mum's outburst and this experience I formed a belief that I had to be perfect to make everybody love me. I can't make people angry. I need to be a people pleaser because if I'm perfect everybody loves me. I need to be the perfect little student. I topped my class in primary school and high school. I studied really hard and I got really good grades. The teachers would love me because I'm perfect. The rest of the students not so much! I copped a lot of bullying because in public schools they don't support academia. Most kids in my area were from troubled homes.

When this strategy didn't work I needed a new one. In my senior year I turned into the party girl and I partied hard, harder than anyone else. I just managed to graduate and gain entry into TAFE, missing out on university because I had screwed up my grades from trying to be cool. In junior high school I had been on track to make it into psychology so I could fulfil my dream of working with people with body image issues, in particular, anorexia and bulimia.

I moved out of home and continued this story of trying to be perfect. I graduated with a diploma of community service, while holding down a full-time job and being the party girl five nights a week. If I could be everything to everyone and do it perfectly, people will love me. Working full-time, studying full-time and out until 3am every night leads to burn out. I was only sleeping a couple of hours a night, living on No-Doz (which ended up being an addiction that I had to kick) and drinking copious amounts. It's no wonder as an adult I got adrenal fatigue because I kept pushing the boundaries.

In my 20s I started bodybuilding so again there's that pursuit of perfection and happiness through the way that I looked. If I looked perfect then everybody would love me.

You can see that I kept searching for this perfectionism and evidence that if I am perfect then everybody would love me. Starting at my origin story of, 'I was abandoned when I was two, therefore there must be something wrong with me'. To fix this, I must be continually searching for perfection. Good grades, the perfect body, people pleasing, best party girl. Constant outsourcing of approval. The only person that had the power to change that was me. Awareness precedes change. Find your origin story and unlock the secret key to self-love.

Do you want to uplevel even further?

Your nurture soul list can be used to create rituals that enhance the feeling of being loved and in flow – allowing the magic to happen.

These rituals get you in the right state. State is that way of being where everything is amazing. We can flip in between states all the time. This can be the state of being tired and exhausted, the state of being flat or the positive state where everything flows.

Going to Coogee is on my nurture list. What state does this give? It allows me time out, to be creative and problem solve. I always come back with brilliant ideas for my own development or business. This ritual of leaving early on Saturday morning, listening to an audiobook on the drive, going to a café to eat raw food cake then spending 4–8 hours on the beach is my life-giving ritual. Listening to the waves, smelling the salt air and watching the seagulls.

Another example is my coffee/salt scrub in the shower followed by lathering myself in coconut oil. I love the smell of coffee and coconut oil! What does this give back to me? It shows that I love, value and respect myself enough to nurture my body. At the end of every day I go across to the park, play ball with Delta my blue cattle dog and listen to music. This is how I sign off my day and know I've finished work. This puts me into a relaxed state. I get to laugh at Delta bouncing around and being over excited by an orange ball.

Your ideal state can be explained as those times where everything flows. Even something as simple as a piece of music can create that state.

If you know what type of state you need to create then you can use things to create this, and they are usually tied to memories. Smells, music, tastes, feel – anything that involves the senses.

I think about the state I was in when I went through a funk with my comps where I failed easy bench lifts that I've done 100 times in the gym. I was stressed out and had been placing so much pressure on myself to succeed (yes that perfectionism stuff again) and I was listening to heavy metal music in between lifts. I had to look at what I was doing and try to create a state that would work, because what I was doing wasn't. So, how did I change my state and go on to break records? I realised it needed to be calm. So my new comp rituals include meditation, leaving plenty of time to get to the venue, not over thinking my lifts, chatting to others and listening to Miley Cyrus's 'The climb'. Those who know me know that is not my usual style but this particular song creates calm in me and that's the state I need to be in. I walk into the gym with my shoulders held back. You'd be surprised what body language does for your physiology.

Now look back at your nurture list and think about those activities and what state you're in when you do them. When can you use these activities to change a state? If I've had a long stressful day, playing with Delta will put me in a happy state. It will change my current state to one that will bring me more of what I want in life – happiness.

Questions from Empowered Eating clients just like you

But Kim, I don't have time!
Schedule even 15 minutes. You will increase productivity 10 times for taking these 15 minutes to yourself. It could be drinking your coffee in silence, while sitting still and being 100% present. It could be curling up with a Hollywood gossip magazine to escape.

But I have so much responsibility...
If you are struggling with time and responsibility, outsource – meal prep, ironing, house cleaning, bookkeeping, business admin, anything to just free up time. The cost of outsourcing is not worth your broken marriage, missing out on that promotion because you can't handle your stress levels or your kids remembering you as the angry raging bull.

What if I can't think of anything?
Think back to your childhood, what did you enjoy then? How did other people show you love? Maybe you snuggled under a doona watching movies on rainy days, maybe Mum took you to get your nails done. Maybe, like me, you loved to rollerblade.

Strategies for your Empowered Eating Toolbox

1. Put your nurture soul list inside the pantry cupboard, so when you feel like you are going to binge, you are reminded to love yourself.

2. Schedule time once a week to show you that you love you, by speaking to yourself in your love language.

3. Talk to your girlfriend, partner or boss about this idea and have accountability.

Chapter 6

Blame elegantly

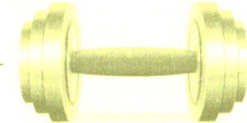

Hold yourself back, or heal yourself back together. You decide.

Brittany Burgunder

Not letting go of the past is like you drinking poison and hoping the other person dies.

When you don't let go of the past, the only person you are hurting is yourself. This pain is causing you to binge eat. You are letting past stories run your present life, forbidding you from having a better future. It's like you are being kept down by invisible shackles. Don't give away your power.

An article on the Tony Robbins website puts it so well:

> *Regardless of what has happened in our lives, we all have one power that can change everything: the power of choice. We cannot choose the events that occur or the circumstances we may find ourselves in, but we can choose what we focus on, what we give meaning to, and what path we will walk down in the future. And it is these three choices, not our conditions, which determine the quality of our lives.*
>
> *Even when you experience a traumatic event, you are given a choice. How will you allow it to impact your life? How are you going to mould it? How are you going to turn your life around? We can allow the stress and uncertainty caused by these events to overwhelm us, or we can transform our lives by making different decisions.*
>
> *Reframing Traumatic Experiences, viewed 20 December 2019, <https://www.tonyrobbins.com/mind-meaning/reframing-traumatic-experiences/>*

Remember Linda from before? She had such a traumatic childhood, she keep soothing emotions from the past with food. By creating her marshmallow suit from emotional eating she was giving away her power. She kept running the same story from the past and not changing the future – only she was dying inside from the poison.

If you are going to blame the past for all the bad, you must also blame it for all the good. Doing this means you get to reframe your story. You get to change your future. Blaming elegantly is looking at the gifts of your childhood trauma. Your trauma gave you some valuable resources and skills. We are going to blame from our soul, with all heartfelt emotion, not just the logical brain.

We will blame consciously.
Blame powerfully.
Blame elegantly.
Blame effectively for all the good and all the bad.
Blame from your soul not the level of your head.

Empowered Eating story time

My biological father was an evil man. He has said and done some pretty horrendous things. Things that I should not have been subjected to growing up. From 13 years onwards I endured trauma that no kid should have and that trauma haunts me to this day.

I soothed my deep-seated pain by binge drinking and binge eating. It helped to numb the memories, it helped push down the anger. I learnt how not to feel emotions. I never let myself feel true happiness as happiness was always taken away from me.

After my first marriage broke down I knew that I couldn't carry that baggage into another relationship. I invested over $30,000 in therapy to get better.

One of the massive turning points was learning how to blame elegantly. To blame effectively for all the good and all the bad. Learning how to turn this pain into a skill. If I didn't go through what I went through, I wouldn't be the coach I am today. I wouldn't have the empathy. I wouldn't have the strategies to teach you.

If I am to blame for all the good, I need to blame him for my drive to prove him wrong. He said I would be in a gutter, and never amount to anything. It drove me to be at the top of my game as a world champion powerlifter and take away silver and gold medals. To have the passion to help others reframe their pain and stop drinking the poison. You don't get to this level of success without dealing with your pain and the poison that is eating you up inside.

If I didn't blame with all of my emotions and feel deeply then I would just be blaming from my head. Blaming from my soul meant feeling complete gratification for all these experiences.

Look at your pain and turn that pain into a skill. Take a really good look at what's gone on in your life. Look at what you have framed as pain and ask yourself what skills you've gained.

For me, I wouldn't be as resourceful, stubborn, driven or as committed as I am. Because I wanted to prove him wrong. I chose this as my driver to be successful and without that one phrase I wouldn't be where I am today, here writing this book to help you. There are so many skills that I've gained from this horrendous situation. I choose to blame elegantly, to blame for all the good and all the bad.

Blame elegantly that you know the opposite. I knew the exact father that I wanted for my future kids. I wanted the exact opposite of what I had seen. I went on 49 dates to find my now husband. I knew that I was going to marry him the day I saw him with his niece and nephews. He was loving, protective, he made them feel safe. He could play and have water fights. He would lay down his life for them. He loves them more than life itself.

Look at your pain. What is hurting you? What skills do you now have as a result of enduring this pain? What have you learnt? Ask yourself what's the learning? What are the positives? What skills have come from this situation that caused pain? What tools has it given me? What are the gifts? I promise you, if you look hard enough like I did, you will find that there are gifts in your pain.

What do you do now, that is the exact opposite to what you experienced? What did you pledge that you will do differently? What will you not tolerate because of what you experienced? How do you stand in your space when things trigger you? What gets your hackles up and you will not put up with at any cost?

For Tanya that is child protection. She was severely beaten as a child for the simplest things, starved daily and screamed at for just being a kid. Her opposite drives her passion to work with kids in child protection. She wants the opposite for these little innocent souls.

Unfortunately as horrible as it is and as hurtful as it is, we have all gone through some form of pain. If we don't look at what skills we have gained from the situation, we will never move forward. We will continue to run the same story and drink the same poison.

By going through this process and journaling these answers you are looking at it differently. It's like you're building a house and we're all looking in from the outside. We know it has a roof and we know it has walls and we know it has a cement floor but I'm looking to the bathroom window and I see a vanity and a shower. You're looking through the kitchen and see cooktops and dishwashers. It is still the same house just a totally different view. By blaming elegantly you have a totally different view.

I want you to trust the process by doing the hard emotional work. I am testifying to you that the hard work is worth it. With a binge eating and binge drinking habit there was no way I could get on world stage and weigh in butt naked, consistently hitting 63kgs. If I still used food to soothe this just wouldn't happen, my lifting would also suffer as I am not fuelling my body right. I want you to really look at your life and move on from the situation. You can be a victor not a victim. Stand on the platform of life with me and take on the world!

I am confident that you will be able to find what gift this situation has given you. I know, if you spend some time meditating and thinking deeply about it you'll be able to find the gifts, because trust me there are gifts. There are gifts in our pain. If you end up crying ugly, cry, tears streaming down your face, mascara running, know that you are exactly where you need to be. This is all part of the healing. Part of letting go. Part of cleansing your body.

Cover the following four steps in the space below or in your journal:

1. Blame for the gifts that you have

_____

2. Blame for the resources you now have emotionally

_____

3. Blame that you know the opposite

_____

4. Blame for the life skills

_____

Do you want to uplevel even further?

Find a way to release this emotion in a creative way. It could be writing poetry, this was especially helpful to me as a teenager. Playing songs that reflect how you feel on an instrument, dance in a way that your soul tells you, to music that talks to you. Some people find drawing cathartic. Take out pencils and paper and draw whatever comes up for you. It could be symbols; it could be using a particular colour that represents your emotions. It could be a group of lines. It could be a postcard you never send. It could look like one of the pictures you drew at three years old. It could be scenic like a storm. The arts, in whichever format can be so healing and an integral part of your process. If any of the above speaks to you, YouTube will help you to get started. Remember it doesn't need to be perfect, just your unique way of releasing.

Questions from Empowered Eating clients just like you

Kim, I can't remember anything from my childhood.
I used to be like this and there are definitely gaps. My brother will mention something from our childhood and I will have no recollection. I started by meditating, using quiet time to just go back to what I could. I always had my journal handy to jot down any memories that came up, the good, the bad and the downright ugly. Find the earliest memory and go from there. It may take days, weeks or even months to piece memories back together. We buried the good and the bad ones as a way to keep us safe as children.

Isn't this saying that their behaviour was ok?
By NO means we are not justifying behaviour and the injustice. We are choosing to stop drinking the poison. I will never condone what happened to me as a child, however, only I had the power to change who drank the poison. By continuing with my destructive behaviour of binge drinking and binge eating then I was the one destroying my life. My biological father was happy living his life, not laying awake at night thinking of the negative impact he has had on his daughter. I had to take 100% responsibility for the way I was reacting, 100% responsibility for the meaning and belief that I had placed on my experiences. I made these experiences mean that I was not worthy, I didn't deserve love, success and happiness. I am responsible for my reactions, my belief system. His behaviour does not mean I am not loveable or cannot be successful. He no longer has that power over me.

What if I lose it emotionally and can't cope?
Please, please I beg you to seek the help of a registered psychologist. It's ok to feel emotions and a psychologist will help you move through the kaleidoscope of emotions that will come up from these memories.

Strategies for your Empowered Eating Toolbox

1. Journal the four blame steps. You can do this for different people in your life.

2. Hold a ceremony of choice to let it go. This could be burning your pages of writing, burying it in the backyard and having a funeral as those parts of you have been laid to rest.

3. Forgive and release. Let it go. You no longer drink poison.

Words on these pages cannot express the full extent of my emotions when I did this activity. I filmed a Facebook live where I was completely raw and emotional. It took three goes to film it as I kept choking up. I have later uploaded it on YouTube as it is very powerful for others to understand the magnitude of facing their fears. You can see it here: https://www.youtube.com/watch?v=FDuVwsD1HjQ&t=156s

Chapter 7

CAR and STONE

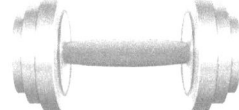

We either make ourselves miserable, or we make ourselves strong. The amount of work is the same.

Carlos Castaneda

Would you believe me if I told you, you are in charge of your life? You get to choose your reaction, your intention and your outcome. Imagine you are lying on your deathbed wishing you hadn't been so miserable and played victim. The last regret I want for you is that you are laying there wishing that you didn't spend so much mental energy on being negative about food and having this ongoing roller-coaster relationship with food.

As Bronnie Ware says in her the book *The Top Five Regrets of the Dying*:

The most common wish of the dying is 'I wish that I had let myself be happier'. Many did not realise until the end that happiness is a choice. They had stayed stuck in old patterns and habits. The so-called 'comfort' of familiarity overflowed into their emotions, as well as their physical lives. Fear of change had them pretending to others, and to their selves, that they were content.

I don't want that for you. I don't want you to be miserable and negative about your life because you emotionally ate every weekend, sending yourself spiralling out of control. I don't want you hating your body. I don't want you avoiding mirrors. I don't want your kids to think that Mum was lifeless and sad. Life is to be lived.

I think we are friends now and I can give you some tough love. Bad things happen to good people, including yourself. You can play victim and eat yourself through a whole jar of Nutella because of what happened to you or you can go out and slay your demons. From the previous chapters we understand how you operate and why you have the thoughts that you do. We know how to blame elegantly for all the good and all the bad. Now it's time to speed forward.

We are going to use a little story to paint the picture.

A CAR is rolling down a mountain creating huge momentum. Much like you are creating the life you want, you are taking responsibility for your world. This is you towards your goal but watch out! You've hit a huge big STONE! A situation has thrown you off your course.

A STONE is stuck. You indulge in stories and excuses as to why you can't have the life that you imagined.

Do you keep driving your CAR knowing you have **Choice**?
Do you take massive **Action** to change the outcome?
Do you take **Responsibility** for your response?

CAR AND STONE

Or do you let the STONE stop your journey by making **Stories** about what happened?
Do you tell yourself it's **Too hard**?
Obfuscate (confuse the issue), never getting to the bottom of what is really holding you back?
Do you believe that you have **No** choice?
Do you make **Excuses** not to change?

Being a CAR can be referred to as being in control of your own destiny and being a STONE is about being stuck, just letting life happen to you.

C Choice
A Action
R Responsibility

S Stories
T Too Hard
O Obfuscation
N No Choice
E Excuses

Living life as a STONE means you are at the mercy of the world around you. You have all types of excuses why you can't do things, why you are not successful. You say things like, 'It's because of the kids', 'It's because I have no money' or 'I don't have time'. These excuses show up in stories like, 'If only you knew what had happened to me, you would understand'. A story is about shifting blame and responsibility from ourselves to things outside our control. Common stories include: 'It's too hard', 'I'm too old', 'I'm too young', 'I'm a woman' and 'I'm not smart enough'.

A story is what you tell yourself to justify why you have the habits and behaviours that you do. There is a feeling of disempowerment, feelings of no other choice, there are no options to change, and there is no control over your position in life. Being stuck by obfuscation, procrastinating, self-pity and excuses.

Driving the CAR is about being in control. If you ever interact with someone who is driving their own car of life, the way they speak will give you hints to their success. Their language will be positive, they will take ownership for their behaviour and they will believe that they are in control of their own journey.

Living like this allows for maximum opportunity and potential to create the outcomes that you are looking for. It will help you make things the way you want them to be. If you dump all the reasons, excuses and stories of why you can't succeed, then you will start driving the car of life and get the results you want.

You will realise there is a choice in every situation in life. You will stop thinking about how bad the situation is, and start choosing whether or not it serves to survive in that story as an excuse as to why you can't change or achieve your goals.

Start taking responsibility for where you are in life. Realise it is possible to make different choices that will take you where you want to go.

It is very easy to live your life as a STONE but it takes courage and action to drive your CAR to success and true happiness.

Empowered Eating story time

For most of my life I had lived as a stone. You have heard parts of my story through this book and could forgive me if I played victim. Playing victim was a strategy that worked, it made people feel sorry for me. I endured some pretty horrible things in my life, my biological father left me so I am unlovable. Enduring domestic violence. Having a stepfather, who every time he looks at me, it is with disgust. Being bullied in high school. My boyfriend committing suicide when I was 17. I have every reason to be a victim and stay stuck. Through most of my teenage and early adulthood I was stuck. Binge drinking and binge eating, smoking, partying, addicted to No-Doz. I was angry at the world. I walked around with a big FU sign on my head. My favourite song was 'Daughter' by Pearl Jam as the chorus had the phrase, 'Don't call me daughter'. I was angry at my biological father for everything that he had done and yet he had the audacity to call me daughter. (I later found out that the song was actually about a girl who was dyslexic). I used attention seeking as a way to prop up my own shattered self-esteem, yet never letting people get close enough to see the real me. I didn't trust men as they either leave or do wrong by me. I only let people see what I wanted them to see. I wasn't authentic, I wasn't real. I wore a mask.

I was a STONE. I ran the same story that I wasn't lovable, it's too hard to get help for my past, it is easier to bury it. I obfuscated telling myself my behaviour wasn't that bad. I had no choice. This was who I was and I couldn't change. Every event that happened to me was an excuse why I couldn't have a better world.

It wasn't until I was 28 that I realised there was a choice. That I could change my past. I could take action through therapy and finally take complete 100% responsibility for my behaviour.

Now I have a life I could only dream of. I have a husband that loves me, a career where I get to change the world, I get to speak on stage inspiring and motivating others, I represent Australia in a sport that I love and I get to write this book for you, Actually I need to reframe my language here. Not *I get to* – *I choose to* because I chose to be a car. Choice Action Responsibility.

Rachel's story

I was coaching Rachel and her STONE story was one of the most interesting ways that we keep ourselves stuck. She was struggling to change her body composition and after some real hard truths about her marriage we discovered that she keeps getting larger so that her husband sees her. It makes her visible. If you think about it, the more visible she is by becoming larger, the more he will actually see her. The current state of her marriage was that he was too engrossed in his work to notice her. She felt invisible in her own marriage. Her story was that *I don't matter to my husband*. It's too hard to be a grown up about this and ask for her needs for attention and affection to be met. She obfuscated that extra body weight wasn't that bad. There was no choice or better way to get his attention. She kept giving me excuses why she couldn't speak up in her own marriage. She even wanted to test him to see if he still loved her regardless of size.

To become a CAR that moves forward she declared that she was choosing to use weight as a very unresourceful way to get her husband's attention. She took action by standing in her space and being completely honest with her husband about what she was doing then asked him for his help and support to get healthy. She admitted to me all she wanted was for her husband to kick her up the butt as that would mean he cared and was giving her attention. She took responsibility for the relationship and booked into couples counselling.

Activity

Now take the time to think about a situation where you are living your life as a STONE. In the space below or in your journal write about the story that you are running in your head. If you're telling yourself it's too hard, obfuscating, confusing the issue and thinking that you have no choice over the situation, what are the excuses you are telling yourself as to why you can't have what you desire?

_____

_____

_____

_____

Now flip the story, and write about what it is going to take to start driving the CAR again.

How am I being stuck like a STONE? What am I telling myself?

_____

What phrases or language do I use that are negative and takes me further from my goal?

_____

How do I obfuscate, procrastinate and/ or self-sabotage?

_____

How is it that I think I have no choice or options?

_____

What excuse do I tell myself and others?

_____

Moving forward, being the driver of the CAR, brainstorm three choices you have.

_____

What actions can you take? Name three.

_____

_____

What responsibilities can you take? Name three.

_____

_____

Do you want to uplevel even further?

Sometimes choice takes a little daydreaming and creativity. Put on some music, light a candle and get writing. Powerlessness and hopelessness comes from a lack of choice. Let's move from this place of stuckness to 100% responsibility by focusing on what you can do not what you can't do. Brainstorm at least 20 choices, and don't worry if some of them seem silly or impossible. There is no judgement here, we are just looking for options. What if you had one million dollars, what would that enable you to do? If you were only given six months to live, what would you do differently that you are not doing today? Now find three that are possible and will lead you to a different outcome to what you are currently getting. Write three massive actions you are going to take and identify three responsibilities you will foster to get to that state you are choosing to live out of.

Questions from Empowered Eating clients just like you

What if my stone won't move?
Go back to Chapter 4 and spend time journaling and meditating on why you have fears around moving forward. What is keeping you safe? Remember as human beings we only do things because we get a reward for it. For example, the reason one of my clients Caitlin couldn't shift weight was that the last time she was successful at shifting weight her sister got jealous, said nasty things and stopped spending time with her.

What if it's the other person's fault?
The only person you can control is yourself and your reaction. You cannot own the other person's behaviour; you can however own yours. Blaming the other person, spending your whole life bitter and twisted about it is like drinking poison and expecting the other person to die. I could 100% blame my father for my drinking problem as a teenager. I could tell the world that I was a failure because of all the traumatic things that happened to me or I could choose to live a better life and take control of my destiny.

What if I can't change anything?
Get 100% radical and think of something so far out of your comfort zone. Living in Queensland growing up on the Sunshine Coast

earning $300 per week, living out of home with no family support, I decided to do something radical. I moved to Uluru. I never looked back; it changed my life forever. I learnt to be brave, pay off my debt and how to chase down my dreams. Moving to the desert was pretty radical.

Strategies for your Empowered Eating Toolbox

1. Look at the shadow side of your life and where you are playing small. Use the Stone analogy and write about where you are being stuck using Stories, Too Hard, Obfuscating, No Choice and Excuse.

2. Own that you want to be a hot red sports car which means that you will say I choose…….. Write about how you will take action and full 100% responsibility.

3. Take one small (or big if you want to catapult change) action in the next 24 hours towards having the life you deserve.

Chapter 8

It's not food, it's me

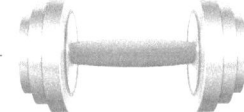

You're not a puppy dog, don't reward yourself with food.

Unknown

This is by far the most impactful quote that I use with my clients. Somewhere in their childhood they were given food as a reward and this behaviour then carries forward into adulthood. Fran had this coding, 'I have had a stressful day at the office, I'll get some takeaway on the way home'. Managing a staff of 20 and being responsible negotiating between stakeholders in government meant that most of her days were stressful. To break this reward cycle she needed to take a different route on the way home to change the environment. We then began investigating where this coding came from. Her mum would take her out for a chocolate sundae when her siblings were mean to her. Food was also a reward when she received good grades at school. Two of Fran's mantras were, 'Feel your emotions don't eat them' and 'To find the treasure, we must first dig through the dirt'. The dirt refers to finding out where the unresourceful behaviour came from in the first place.

This is only one example of how you were coded in childhood, and we are going to dig deeper to find the patterns, stories and old beliefs around food.

Some of these patterns are centred around holding on to painful events, feelings, hurt and shame around things that happened in childhood, especially in puberty when as females we gain breasts and our body shape changes. When you are made to feel ashamed about your body you will keep yourself safe by resorting to food. Carrying the shame from childhood impacts every area of your life and by doing so it impacts your confidence. If we don't shine a torch into these dark areas you are at a high risk of sabotaging your progress.

We are going to forgive the people who did wrong by you, coded you in an unresourceful way and also forgive yourself for continuing the same coding as an adult. Through coaching I quite often discover that clients are still running childhood strategies in response to adult problems as this was what they were taught as a child. We will release and forgive so that you can be free to choose a different response. When you choose not to forgive then you are staying stuck like a stone and you'd be more accurate calling your lack of forgiveness self-punishment. We are learning a new strategy of self-permission, working with the unconscious part of you that likes to sabotage your results. Changing from the space of self-punishment to self-permission is the most powerful antidote to old behaviours.

By forgiving from a soul level you can open up the doors of possibility to other areas of your life. It is surprising the amount of emotional energy and head miles that goes into guilt around food. When you don't have this constant cloud over your head, you can be free to see other opportunities, you will take bigger leaps into the direction of your dreams. For Katherine that meant starting her own career coaching business. For so many years, she had been consumed with food, what types of food to eat, when not to eat, to only eat healthy things in front of other people and bingeing in private. There was a whole host of shame about not being able to stick to a diet and a fear of being visible. Until we worked through all these head miles to uncover *why* she was sabotaging her results she didn't have the mental capability to start her new business.

There may be some phrases that you can think of immediately that coded you? Were you told to eat everything on your plate? There are starving kids in Africa? If you don't eat all your dinner you won't get dessert? To be skinny and popular you must only eat salad?

We are all the products of our coding. Here's an explanation from a research paper on parental influence on eating behaviour:

> *Although children possess an innate ability to self-regulate their energy intake, the extent to which they exercise this ability is determined by environmental conditions: for example, offering large food portions, calorically rich, sweet or salty palatable foods; the use of controlling feeding practices that pressure or restrict eating; and the modelling of excessive consumption can all undermine self-regulation of energy intake in children.*
>
> Savage, JS, Fisher, JO & Birch, LL 2007, 'Parental influence on eating behaviour: conception to adolescence', *Journal of Law, Medicine & Ethics*, vol. 35(1), pp. 22–34.

Our childhood coding of either overfeeding or underfeeding has a huge impact on our relationship with food. It stems from the adults that taught us.

If these stories are not dealt with, you will stay the same. That means you will be this exact same shape next year. The definition of insanity is doing the same thing over again and expecting different results.

We are going to look back over your childhood and find out where you learnt certain things about food, body image and negative self-talk

Lucy's story

Coding from teenage years have such strong anchors around body image and food. If you are struggling to find your coding this is a really great place to start. Lucy and I had a conversation about why she was resistant to meal prep:

Lucy: I am often afraid of eating and that is why I don't put effort into meal prep.

Kim: What is it about eating that scares you?

Lucy: Eating has made me overweight... And my brain seems to cut out all the important other stuff and just shortens it to this. My logic knows that isn't right but this is the thought I became aware of today.

Kim: So what is the truth behind this?

Lucy: Eating does not make me overweight... eating too many calories does. It just seems odd to me to even have that thought.

Kim: However, your unconscious brain gave you that thought for a reason. There must be some element to this statement that it believes.

Lucy: Ok… I think it comes from this. When I was a teen to early 20s the girls that were skinny and popular you never saw them eat. If you went to lunch with them they would have like two chips and coffee. At parties they never ate the food.

Kim: So to be happy, successful and accepted you must not eat?

Lucy: That's what my unconscious brain believes. Time to journal, forgive and release!

Kim: Awareness precedes change. When you understand where these thoughts and beliefs come from you can rewrite them to something resourceful. Changing how you respond differently in the future. A huge well done on finding the origin story!

Empowered Eating story time

My relationship with food in my teenage years was terrible and disordered. I would eat two rice cakes per day as I saw in *Dolly* magazine that rice cakes had very few calories. The teenager in me twisted that to mean that was how you lose weight. Having 70 calories per day resulted in frequent fainting. I was 43kg but thought I was fat. If I did overeat as my biology was overriding me, I would purge with laxatives. I just wanted to be loved and accepted.

Emily copped so much bullying for reaching puberty earlier than everyone else. The girls in her grade teased her because she was the first to start menstruating. She developed large breasts and the boys would ask for piggyback rides so that they could look down her top. Poor Emily didn't even realise this was their strategy until she was older. As her coach I could see the physical manifestation of this story. Her posture was poor, she walked with hunched shoulders to hide her big breasts. All this unwanted attention made her feel unsafe, all she wanted to do was hide.

Sara was fat-shamed by her mother at 10. Her mother took her to weight loss groups and constantly belittled her for overeating. This meant that she would sneak food that her brothers were allowed. This started a lifelong cycle of secret eating.

Katherine grew up in a family of 13 kids so everything had to be shared. This included the 1L soft drink bottle with 13 straws and backwash. When she started working as a teenager she would buy and hide food so that she wasn't forced to share with her siblings. Enter a lifetime of hiding food, including never eating in front of her husband.

My first boss as a 13-year-old took me to the storeroom and told me to sit on his knee. I felt sick to my stomach that something was going to happen. I was aware enough to know I wasn't safe. Thankfully another employee walked in to get the mop, stopping whatever was going to happen. That night I binged on a block of cookies and cream chocolate. This is just another story filed in Kim's brain that men are not safe. Yes I know 13 is illegal to be working but I begged my Mum to let me. I wanted my own money and to be independent. I associated being alone with being unsafe. When I moved out of home and my flatmates left me alone in the house I would binge on their food as I didn't feel safe. My origin story is where my boss told me to sit on his lap and that night bingeing from feeling unsafe and to get rid of that icky feeling in my stomach.

Activity

Look at the following questions and think back to where in your past this showed up. Take out your journal and write as much as you can remember, or circle those that apply below and add your own too. Put everything down in your journal or on this page.

Release the blocks. Forgive. Let it go. Become neutral about it.

1. Forgive for all the negative self-talk and body shame. Here are some examples that you may have said to yourself. Write them all down.
- I am fat
- Look at those tuckshop arms
- Squeezing fat rolls
- I have so much cellulite on my butt
- If I lost weight I would be happier
- _____

2. Forgive for all the unhealthy diets, training and disordered habits. Anything unhealthy that you have tried including:
- Lemon detox
- Fat blaster tablets
- Shake diet
- Laxatives
- Overtraining
- Starvation
- Atkins
- Drugs
- Alcohol
- No-Doz
- 1200 calories or less
- _____

3. Forgive all the people who modelled unhealthy behaviour. These may include:
- Mum who snuck food
- Being taken to weight loss groups as a kid
- Celebrities that modelled thin is in – I think of Kate Moss
- Women who starve themselves post-baby for the red carpet
- Instagram models
- Mum that won't eat in front of kids
- Rewarding with food
- Hearing others negative self-talk

- Schools who weigh kids
- You must eat everything on your plate or you won't get dessert
- You can't leave the table until you have finished everything on your plate
- There are starving kids in Africa that are dying
- Sweating is wrong
- _____

4. Forgive all the people for nasty, mean or inappropriate things said, such as:
- The inappropriate uncle
- Being teased for getting your menstrual cycle early
- Boys harassing over seeing your breasts
- Males staring at your breasts
- Being called fatty boomba
- You're too sexy
- You're too fat
- You're too skinny
- You're too muscular (this was all from one client)
- Boys asking for piggy back so can look down top
- You are a whale
- Horrible jokes
- Making grunting sounds
- _____

5. Forgive all the shame and disrespectful actions towards your body like:

- Sleeping with guys for attention
- Drinking far too much
- Drug abuse
- Eating cotton wool to feel full
- Hiding in baggy clothing
- Poor posture from having breasts that were noticed
- _____

Do you want to uplevel even further?

Talk to a close girlfriend about her experiences growing up to help her heal. I spoke with a friend about what body image was like for her growing up. She had learned that to be popular at school she had to be skinny. Where did she learn this? She was hanging out with her older sister and her best friend and they were talking about diets and the only way the popular girls were going to like them was if they were following the lemon detox diet. The friend of the sister encouraged my girlfriend to diet for the first time (she was 11!!) so that she could be part of the popular group. The story and belief that came out of this was that you must diet to be popular.

Questions from Empowered Eating clients just like you

What if my mum modelled healthy behaviour to me?
You are very lucky that your mum has a healthy relationship with food. There may have been other influences growing up as to why you may have disordered feelings towards food. A good place to start is the media and their portrayal of body image.

What if the shame is overwhelming?
If shame runs deep from trauma, I am saying as your coach that seeing a psychologist is the best path for you. We need you to heal so that you can have a healthy relationship with food.

What if I feel funny talking to myself in the mirror?
It will feel strange and that is ok. Practice makes it easier. It is common to feel uncomfortable hearing and receiving compliments. This makes it even more important for you to do this work. The reason for my confidence is that I speak so highly of myself in the mirror. I feel safe with attention from the opposite sex because I am kind to myself and I am familiar with compliments. I can stand in my space and set boundaries if it becomes too much.

Strategies for your Empowered Eating Toolbox

1. Write a forgiveness letter to yourself for all the wrong actions and words you've said to yourself.

2. Write a forgiveness letter to the bullies, Mum or the creepy uncle.

3. Change the way you speak to yourself if you have learnt it is not safe to be visible and you are using food as a protective shield. You unconsciously believe the unwanted body fat keeps you safe and helps you not stand out or receive unwanted attention. Try saying these statements to yourself:
   • I am enough
   • I love and approve of myself
   • I am worthy.

By saying at least one of the above statements in the mirror every day I am getting you to become comfortable with hearing compliments. This makes you feel safer preventing you from sabotaging your own behaviour.

Here's the link to a bonus video on the subject from when I spoke about this on Facebook:
https://facebook.com/234947206582487/videos/2512825295703718/

Chapter 9

Life detox

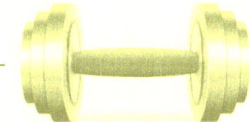

> Anxiety arises from not being able to see the whole picture. If you feel anxious, but are not sure why, try putting your things in order.
>
> Marie Kondo

Cluttered space, cluttered mind. A clear mind doesn't resort to emotional eating as a way of coping from the overwhelm.

Your environment is a direct reflection of your mindset. When your environment becomes clear, your mind becomes clear. Decluttering your home as a way of breaking through your bingeing has other benefits. By creating physical space in your home it opens up space for abundance to come into your life. It increases energy as you feel lighter walking into a room and not seeing clutter. You could also make money while selling all your unwanted toys, gifts and clothes.

Purging these items helps you let go of the past, including physical items that anchor in old feelings of failure like a failed relationship. Samantha's ex-husband gave her a dinner set for her 40th birthday. She was so disheartened as she wanted a ring for her 40th, not a dinner set. He had gifted the dinner set after she saw it in Myer and said it was nice. It was a passing comment, not a request for him to buy it. She didn't want the constant reminder of the fact that he never really understood her, even when she told him that she wanted a ring as her gift. It was such an emotional release to sell that dinner set and she brought a ring with the money!

What emotional anchors are around your house that keep you anchored in past memories that you need to detox? One of the only three gifts my biological father gave me was a 2cm tall cotton woven worry doll worth maybe $5 max. On the same day I saw him buy his friend a 1L bottle of rum and 1L bottle of bourbon worth over $100. This anchored in how little I was worth to him. I don't need that negative emotional energy of *I am not worthy according to my biological father* so I threw it in the garbage. You can't attract positivity into your life if you are still surrounded by the negative.

When you have a higher standard for yourself by removing all broken and damaged goods in your home you will start to see that you are worthy of nice things and will hold yourself to a higher standard. The flow on effect is that you will no longer compromise or take crap in other areas of your life.

Decluttering overdue bills and paperwork is a big one. It is highly symbolic, and it shows the universe that you are moving towards the new version of you, one that pays your bills on time. What other items in your house are showing evidence of the old you that will be highly symbolic to the universe once you have changed? It could be the ice cream bowl that you always use when you are on your binge frenzy. The one where you crush up chocolate biscuits, add it to the ice cream and then drown it with copious amounts of melted Nutella. You will be constantly reminded of your failures, embarrassment and generally feel crap about yourself if you don't remove these items.

You would be surprised at the evidence of overeating and excess calorie consumption due to chaos.

> *Participants in the chaotic kitchen condition and the out-of-control mindset condition consumed more cookies (103 kcal) than did participants who were in the in-control mindset condition (38 kcal).*
>
> Vartanian, L, Kernan, KM & Wansink, B 2016, 'Clutter, Chaos, and Overconsumption: The Role of Mind-Set in Stressful and Chaotic Food Environments', *Environment and Behaviour*, vol. 49 (2), pp. 215–223.

Do you need further motivation?

> When people declutter and organise their homes, they often lose weight as a natural by-product, without even trying!
> **Melissa Howell, Beautiful Life and Home**

In the last chapter we started decluttering some of the emotional coding that we learnt from childhood. We are going to go deeper this chapter into other areas that can be cluttering your mind and making it difficult for you to stop bingeing.

By the end of this chapter you will have a plan that shows you how to declutter emotionally and physically.

Lucy's story

Do you remember Lucy from earlier and how she was evicted from her long-term home? This is her story about decluttering and the impact on her mental health.

After a move from a large home to a small house on a farm I struggled with all the stuff. We had our belongings everywhere. Nothing had a home or a permanent place. I would constantly walk into the room feeling overwhelmed and not know where to start. I struggled with my daily routines and rituals as my house was so cluttered and messy. I was using food as a way of soothing the overwhelm. After a session with Kim she suggested that I start in one room, in one corner and work my way through it all systematically. For me this was the living room. I unpacked one box at a time and removed so much clutter. The amount of joy and confidence this one small step gave me was more than I expected. The shift in my mindset from overwhelm to 'I've got this' was like magic.

Declutter. Declutter. Declutter. And just when you think you've decluttered enough... Declutter some more. Your mind and physical space holds onto too much! It's not needed! Release the crap!

Empowered Eating story time

Decluttering under couches, in wardrobes and old clothes I've found money – it's hidden in all kind of places. I also tackled my bank statements, to see where I was spending money for no apparent reason. I rang my phone company and asked them to review what I was paying per month, so they've knocked $55 off the price per month and doubled my data. Next was the insurance company. I combined my insurance policies with one company and have saved over $300 per year. I cancelled my dating app subscription because I wasn't using it! I wanted to meet guys the old fashion way. This saved over $40 per month and I'd been paying this for seven months. I have sold

30 items from my wardrobe making a nice $600 back from designer clothes that are too baggy after shifting 9kgs. I'm about to call and cancel a charity payment I make per month because the charity doesn't spark me with joy – I'm sure I can quote Marie Kondo when I call them right? I have avoided doing this for at least a year out of guilt. But when I see the money out of my bank account each month it makes me feel guilty. I'll cancel that today too.

Where to start

The following lists and the examples given are only to kickstart your memory, and help you start to declutter both emotionally and physically. It's definitely not extensive.

Emotional:

- Stories from parents about food which we touched on in the last chapter. Just check there is nothing left
- Coding around food and phrases you may have heard growing up, e.g. eat everything on the plate
- Money stories – money and food are closely linked. Did you come from a family of scarcity with money and you have the same mentality with food so when there is free food you must take it?
- Money coding, e.g. you may have heard that money is dirty, or told that money doesn't grow on trees
- Shame around yo-yo dieting. This could be the disapproving look from your mother about the new diet you are following
- Shame around letting old you go. Clients have a lot of shame around getting married and not taking care of their appearances
- Shame around being visible. This could have been the boys leering at you on the school bus
- Shame for not setting boundaries and letting people take advantage of you

- Shame for not speaking up. About injustice you witnessed or not speaking up when your needs are not being met
- Shame around puberty being made fun of as your breast bounced in sport
- Shame from religious authorities, to never outshine others as this is not godly, spiritual people can't be rich
- Shame for being different, you had a different way of relating to others making you different
- Shame around being sexy. Confidence and sex appeal can be bullied out of you by other females
- Forgiveness for nasty self-talk, for all the nasty things you have said to yourself
- Forgiveness letters to Mum for any of your food coding or parenting style
- Forgiveness letters to Dad for being absent or never telling you that he is proud of you
- Forgiveness letter to family that could be siblings or cousins and extended family
- Forgiveness letters to bully at school who made your first year hell
- Forgiveness letters to teachers for telling you that you will not amount to anything
- Forgiveness letters for nasty diets – cabbage soup, lemon detox, so many!
- Forgiveness letters to ex-partners for the way they treated you
- Cheating, knowing it's not all you when your partner cheats
- Break ups, owning responsibility for your bit. We can all take responsibility for our relationship breaking down
- Lessons learnt from ex-partners.

Overall declutter:

- Fix/ declutter things that aggravate you like range hood lightbulb that doesn't work

- Declutter broken items, toys, kitchen items, everything
- Declutter items that no longer suit your lifestyle. I emptied my closet of all my hippy beach wear as that's not me anymore
- Declutter anything that is not you – I decluttered all my bodybuilding posters
- Declutter reminders of past failures – I threw out old business cards
- Declutter obligation items like the tea cosy my grandma gave me
- Declutter items that don't serve you. I have VR goggles that came free with my phone that I need to sell
- Declutter unwanted gifts. Jewellery falls into this category, it's such a personal thing
- Declutter unused expensive items. I had a pair of Doc Martens from the 90s that I never wore, in my 20s they were so expensive
- Declutter items that you'll use 'one day'. I might use that piping bag and cake decorating accessories… *Kim you never bake*
- Declutter items of old relationships. I destroyed my wedding photos
- Declutter items of business failures. I threw out my old business cards of the first time I worked for myself
- Declutter MLM that didn't work. For me this was Amway
- Declutter friends that don't serve. I removed energy vampires from my life
- Declutter old client files – anything past seven year's old needs to be shredded
- Declutter your computer – any old folders, files and documents
- Declutter your phone/ notifications. How many apps do you have that you don't use? For me it's also photos. Too many photos of my dog Delta, trying to get that perfect shot with her ears up
- Declutter paperwork/ old bills. I had a shredding morning, getting rid of all paperwork

- Declutter things that need repair – heels either go to the shoe doctor or in the bin
- Declutter office desk – this one I need to do regularly
- Declutter purse and handbag of all those damn old receipts. File them for tax or just throw them
- Declutter non-working appliances. To be truthful I will never get around to fixing them
- Declutter emails – for me this is still a work in progress
- Declutter Facebook/ Instagram. Remove friends that are negative or don't align with your values.

Declutter home environment:

- Declutter kid's toys
- Declutter CDs/Books/DVDs
- Declutter knick-knacks
- Declutter storage room
- Declutter laundry
- Declutter the junk drawer
- Declutter garage
- Declutter outside storage
- Declutter supplements
- Clean your car
- Clean the glove box
- Clean the boot
- Declutter under bed
- Ditch worn out underwear
- Ditch stretched/ faded/ torn clothes
- Declutter costume jewellery
- Declutter old make-up/ vanity
- Declutter out of date medicine
- Declutter dining table
- Declutter clothes that don't fit
- Declutter shoes
- Declutter pantry

- Declutter Tupperware/ no lids
- Clean fridge.

Do you want to uplevel even further?

Take before and after photos and tag me with #empoweredeatingmindset so we can all celebrate your success. If you are ultra-brave and need the accountability you can share a pic of the 'junk room' in your house, the one that will take several weekends to get through. There is nothing like public accountability to leverage action.

Questions from Empowered Eating clients just like you

What if I feel resistant?
Find one thing to let go of. You will have excuses like, 'I might need it one day'. When was the last time you used it? Or maybe it was a gift. It is still clutter causing you ill feelings and guilt. Get rid of it so there isn't the reminder. It may not be your style or align with the new version of you. You have permission to upgrade and leave reminders of the old you behind.

But I have a pretty clean house...
My house is like this as my husband is OCD about cleanliness. We still have that one shelf in the office that needs constant attention, the garage that needs monthly clean outs and a pantry where the things at the back are past their use-by date. Oh, and my gym bag that collects things.

Strategies for your Empowered Eating Toolbox

1. Create a list of the things that you are going to declutter or alternately download the lists from the bonus section www.transformationsbykim/bookbonuses

2. Commit to doing one thing every week to declutter your house. I don't expect you to declutter everything at once as that would be overwhelming and you will just procrastinate.

3. Take before and after photos to tag me on social media.

You can download your free checklist at: www.transformationsbykim/bookbonuses

Chapter 10

Strawberry friends and chocolate friends

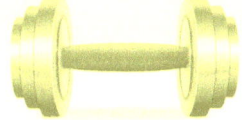

Show me your friends and I'll show you your future.

Unknown

If you are surrounded by unhealthy people your habits will reflect those that you spend time with. You will find yourself eating KFC because they were too lazy to find healthier alternatives.

Here's the harsh truth:

Nicholas Christakis and James Fowler examined the data set from the Framingham Heart Study, one of the largest and longest running health studies ever. According to their results, if a friend of yours becomes obese, you yourself are 45 percent more likely than chance to gain weight over the next two to four years. If your friend is obese or a friend of a friend is obese, that changes your perception of what is an acceptable body size and your behaviour changes accordingly.

Now I am not saying, go around and break up with all your friends because they are overweight, just be aware of their behaviours and how that is influencing you. You are going to need to be really strong. When they order dessert, you need to say no. When they want to catch up over wine, you will need to say no. Being hyper aware of their behaviours and their influence is one strategy, another is upgrading your Tribe, one by one. Spending more time with people who lift you higher. Using the analogy of your hand to count your friends, if you replace the most versatile, the thumb with an upgraded friend then you will grasp your goals better.

'You're the average of the five people you spend the most time with' is a quote attributed most often to motivational speaker Jim Rohn. There's also the 'show me your friends and I'll show you your future' derivative.

Whichever you've heard, the intent is the same. Audit the people around you. Make sure that you're spending time with people who are in line with what you want for your own life

Are you hanging with strawberry friends or chocolate friends?

In life you will find your friendship group can be divided into two groups. Ones that lift you higher and ones that will try and drag you down.

STRAWBERRY FRIENDS AND CHOCOLATE FRIENDS

I like to call them strawberry friends and chocolate friends. Strawberry friends are the encouraging, supportive type of your journey and your choice to compete, lift and train hard with. On the other hand, chocolate friends are those who tell you, missing one session at the gym won't hurt…

The more you surround yourself with strawberry friends the more supported you will be. These are the friends that will catch up with you for a walk or a workout session at the gym and not disregard your choices to live a healthy lifestyle. One of the reasons I have my Tribe and our Empowered Eating Skype Class is so that everyone feels supported and they can make friends with people who are on the same mission as them.

Chocolate friends can also be found in your family. The mother-in-law that says, 'Can't you forget your diet today?' or the partner who says, 'Do you really need to go to the gym? Stay and cuddle'. Going out and socialising there will be more chocolate friends because it's human nature to want our peers to justify our choices. If your friend is indulging in cocktails they will want you to join in so they don't feel guilty.

Stay strong! Plan your food and drinks before going out. Be a little more skimp at breakfast and lunch so you can enjoy treats. I'm going to coffee with my clients this weekend and I will be enjoying raw food cake. It has 30g of fat!! This means no eggs, chia seeds or yogurt that day but it's the price I pay for indulging in raw food cake. Make it fit and enjoy it!

Take a look at your list of friends and see which category they fit into. Remember, we are the sum of the five people that we spend time with, so choose your friends wisely. It's the law of averages.

When you spend time with positive-minded strawberry friends who are successful and believe in taking responsibility for their lives, you will be inspired to do the same. On the flip side, hanging out with chocolate friends who have a pessimistic view on life, will eventually bring you down, no matter how positive you are.

Take the time to reflect on your list and take a deeper look at the strawberry friends. What is it about them that you like? What qualities do they have that you have or would like to have? How do they lift you up? What are their positive attributes and values?

It's important to point out that I'm not recommending you go out and sever relationships with all your chocolate friends. However, it's worth considering reducing the amount of contact you have with people who are not helping (and may even be hindering) you on your journey to become a better person. If someone is seriously bringing you down, you will likely be better off without their influence in your life. When you are stuck in relationships which are not elevating you and are having the opposite effect, you cannot be the best you can be for yourself or for others.

Melanie's story

I was coaching Melanie and she was drinking every weekend, which is not conducive to changing your body composition and getting lean. After asking further questions I discovered she was the only one in her friendship group that went to the gym. I had an honest chat with her and said this journey is going to be increasingly difficult because of who you spend time with and their choice in activities. They provide you with one of the six core needs as a human being which is connection. How can you find connection elsewhere in your life? She thought about the people in the gym and one of the trainers had spoken about her dragon boating team. Melanie knows my analogy of strawberry friends and chocolate friends and how by changing just one can help you grasp your goals. She decided to be brave and ask the trainer if they needed any more people on her dragon boating team. They did – and now she has a whole community of strawberry friends.

Empowered Eating story time

In my Facebook group that I have for all of my clients, one of the Tribe members made a great distinction. She stated that she needs to become her own strawberry friend and speak to herself in a kinder way. Her words were, 'I need to listen to Strawberry Alesha more than Chocolate Alesha who berates and puts me down'. Ask yourself are you being your own strawberry friend?

Jamie said when she did this activity it created a greater appreciation for her strawberry friends and the impact that they have on her life. She is going to celebrate her strawberry friends more. They have positive qualities that she wants more of in her life

Do you want to uplevel even further?

Figure out what each of your strawberry friends' love language is and speak to them in their love language to create a deeper connection. Even better, you can explain to them the concept of love languages or give them a copy of Gary Chapman's book. To inspire them and be a strawberry friend who lifts them higher you can talk about what you have learnt in this book. Not only does this inspire and encourage them to grow, it also cements in your brain the concepts of this book. When you teach someone else what you are learning, it helps you recall and remember information that you have learnt.

Questions from Empowered Eating clients just like you

What if I only have chocolate friends?
Brainstorm places that you can meet new friends. A fun game I have played with my clients is listing from A to Z different places that you can meet people.

Here's our list. Feel free to add more!

- Archery
- Book store
- Camping
- Dog Park, dragon boating
- Entertainment (shows/comedy)
- Flip out
- Game (sport)
- Hiking
- Ice hockey/ skating
- Jumping (trampoline)
- Kiting, kayaking
- Languages, lake walk,
- Museum, master classes
- Nude painting
- Observatory
- Paddle boarding
- Quilting
- Rock climbing, rollerblading
- Sailing, segway
- Tenpin bowling / TunzaFun
- University (short courses)
- Volunteering
- Water skiing
- Xtreme sport
- Yoghurt land
- Zoo

Strategies for your Empowered Eating Toolbox

1. Look at your list of friends and categorise them accordingly. I ended up creating a group in my phone called strawberry friends. When I get a free moment they are the ones I message as the relationships worth nurturing. If I have a free weekend coming up, I message them to go out for coffee or a walk.

2. Ask yourself, what values do these friends have and what values would you like to enhance in your own life? My husband is my strawberry friend. He values cleanliness and his way of being has definitely rubbed off onto me. He has systems for everything. I now have a system for paying my bills.

3. Identify how you can spend more time with these friends.

Chapter 11

You are a shero

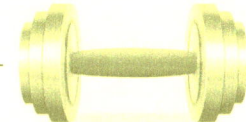

The hero's journey is inside of you; tear off the veils and open the mystery of yourself.

Joseph Campbell

To be binge-free forever you are going to go on your own shero journey. You can be the hero of your own life. There will be times when you slip up. There will be setbacks. However, you are going to get back up and chase your dreams.

You will receive a call to action, to change this bingeing cycle forever and hopefully this book has been a sign from the universe that now is your time to shine and you are ready for the next step.

By understanding your shero journey you can eliminate yo-yo dieting as you will view your behaviour differently.

If you are repeating the journey of weight shifting, you can identify the skills and resources that you have to do it again. It can feel like you are floundering and stuck, stumbling through the dark repeating the same mistakes. By identifying the skills and resources you have within, it helps you get out of your own way and find a solution.

The story of your shero's journey is based on the book *The Hero with a Thousand Faces* by Joseph Campbell. The book describes the steps of the hero's journey, which is really a universal journey that we all take in our lives during times of change and challenges. The story has been depicted in books and films famously and many times over, and we are drawn to it and connect with it as the elements are embedded deep in our psyche.

> The cave you fear to enter holds the treasure you seek.
> **Joseph Campbell**

We are going to plug your story into the hero's journey so you know what your next step should be. What dragons you need to slay. What is on the other side of the cave. How you can evoke hope and create an action plan.

The journey is divided into four main parts:

- Hear the call
- Engage in your journey
- Reset yourself
- Own the new settings.

Activity

1. The first step is to read over the whole journey and think about where you are now.
2. Grab your journal to write about any insights that surface.
3. Answer the questions that follow in the spaces below or in your journal.

Stage 1: The ordinary world
This is groundhog day where you have the same problem, year in year out. You're happy playing average. This was me in 2004, size 16, eating only takeaway and drinking every night. Describe what it was like for you here?

What positives did you give up being here?

___

Stage 2: Call to adventure
Awakened by something, it might be a health scare or your kids pleading you to do something. The doctor told me I was overweight. Realising there is a life beyond this. You are called to do something. The louder the call the closer you will get to the next step.

When were you called to action?
What did you hear?

___

Stage 3: The refusal of the call
Refusal of the call important part of the journey as this will show your commitment to the journey. The biggest fear in this space is of the unfamiliar. I don't know what this will look like, how do I need to change, what if I'm not good enough? It's based on insecurities and unconscious belief systems. You will usually refuse three times because of time or power. It's not the right time, I don't have time to track my food. Power can be money, not good enough or not

sure if it is going to work for me. I had all of these fears when I ran my own business for the first time.

How many times have you said no? Describe them.
___

Along the journey you will have a token or a best friend who will make you feel protected. It might be your husband, a strawberry friend or some symbol/ token. For me it's my grandfather's sapphire ring. I touch that and I know that I have the strength to keep going. As human beings we are more inclined to do something for someone else than for ourselves.

Who is the strawberry friend or token?
___

Stage 4: Meeting the mentor
In this stage you've had enough of a problem and need to do something about it. Now is the time. You look for a mentor or trusted advisor. It could be someone you know like a colleague, a coach that you employ to help you, a book or even someone from afar like Arnold Schwarzenegger. This person has been on this journey already and can guide you on the path. They have the magic, the skills, wisdom that you want. They have the essence of what you are looking for.

Who is that person to you?
___

Stage 5: Crossing the first threshold
This is where the journey of self-discovery really begins. Life will never be the same, you have new habits and ways of beings. You say no to that second glass of wine or bring your lunch to work

every day. Instead of having chocolate every day, you eat chocolate only every second day. It can be confusing in here; people use words like macros and conditioning sessions. It's so unfamiliar and uncomfortable. It could be quitting your job to pursue happiness.

What looks different in this world for you right now?

___

Stage 6: Test. Allies. Enemies.
You're so excited in this world. You know the call is strong and this is your purpose however there are going to be tests, allies and enemies. This is where you will learn what you are really made of. Your thinking is going to change, you will face the enemy of self-doubt, the mini me that throws up stories of the past where you have failed.

What challenges have you faced?

___

You will rely on your mentor here to support you. You will draw strength from this person. They will teach you that you have everything inside you. Instead of leading with your logic brain they will teach you to trust your gut, to fall in love with the mission and then finally lead with your brain.

What has your mentor taught you?

___

Stage 7: The innermost cave
This is the realisation stage where you know that you must face your greatest fear or obstacle or you will go back to the average world. You question why you are doing this. Your friends may not be around at this stage and you feel all alone. You need to make a very tough decision.

What do you need to face to be the hero of your own journey?
_____

Stage 8: The final ordeal
This is battle time! You've hit rock bottom and by overcoming this you will have the power and tools to overcome anything. Everything is put on the line. For me it was meeting my biological father who scared the crap out of me, yet I knew that if I didn't do it then I would continue to binge for the rest of my life. If I can face the fear of a violent evil man who is capable of anything then I can face any fear in my life. Everything else is puny in comparison! Break through the thing that you fear the most, for a life that bears the biggest rewards.

What ordeals have you faced?
How were they life changing?
What tools and resources do you have now that are unbreakable?
What looks different in this world for you right now?

_____

_____

Stage 9: The reward, what you have come for
This is the reward, the success, the inner change. You've become your own hero. You are proud of who you have become and all self-doubt is gone. Sometimes it is underwhelming as you have changed into this person and the goal was actually to be expected as you have worked so hard for this. I had this feeling when I won silver at my first Worlds for powerlifting. It was like I already expected it as that was what I had come for.

Who are you because of your ordeal?
How much work did you put in to overcome this?

What learnings are you ready to bring home?

_____

_____

Stage 10: The road back

This path is not smooth sailing just yet, you're faced with bad habits, temptations, dark past, addictions, ex-partners, just to name a few challenges. What have you learnt that you can apply to the real world? It could be saying no catching up with your ex because you know deep down that you are not that person anymore.

Can you pre-empt the challenges for this stage?
What tools and strategies can you implement to overcome these obstacles when faced again?
What have you learnt from your journey to share with others?

_____

_____

Stage 11: Returning home

Sorry to be the bearer of bad news there is more work to be done! This stage you will be challenged by others on your thoughts and beliefs. People like sameness and you may start to stand out from the crowd. They won't like it and will try and bring you back down. The best advice here is to walk the walk and talk the talk, follow through with everything that you have learnt, be that example to others. Lead from love not ego.

How will you lead by example?

_____

Stage 12: Return with the elixir

At this final stage you have a realisation from sharing and helping others. You know that you have a legacy to leave behind, even if it's just for your kids. You have the experience and the knowledge to educate others. It is your calling to have an impact on the world. It's important that this part of the journey is shared with friends, children, family and the world so you don't resort back to old beliefs and behaviours. It cements your new world. For me this is every fibre of my being. To touch, move and inspire women to have an empowered relationship with food so that they are free to be the woman they are designed to be. At this stage you will realise that you had all the tools and resources already inside you.

How will you share your journey?
Will you use a social platform?
How will you leave a legacy?

Sasha's story

Sasha's story is an example of the shero's journey in action:

Stage 1: Describe what it was like for you here.
I was bingeing out of control, people pleasing and in a yo-yo cycle of dieting. I was not using contraception and wanted to fall pregnant however I had dieted so hard that I damaged my hormones. I knew something needed to change.

What positives did you give up being here?
There was no self-love and a constant restrictive attitude towards food.

Stage 2: When was your call-to-action?
I met Kim at a seminar. I was hearing other girls' experiences and then seeing Kim standing in front of everyone strong healthy and confident even though she had been through something similar as I had with yo-yo dieting. I was overwhelmed and wanted this.

What did you hear?
Initially I needed to let everything sink in. The first step was changing jobs from a toxic environment. After six months at the new job I reached out to Kim. I had the headspace and was ready for her to teach me all the tools that I needed to be in control of my bingeing and have a healthy relationship with food.

Stage 3: How many times did you say no?
The first time was the day that I met Kim, I was so overwhelmed and scared. It took me approximately six months to reach out. I fell pregnant after six months of working with Kim because my hormones were balanced and my emotional state was stable. After my baby was born my world changed. I was trying to get back on track but I used my child as an obstacle. It took me until my little one turned two to wake up and realise this is not what I envisaged for myself and it's time to be accountable again.

Who is the strawberry friend or token?
Kim keeps me accountable my husband supports me and also keep me accountable. My son is my big reason why.

Stage 4: Who is the mentor for you?
Kim – her story is raw, amazing and inspiring. She is real, true and authentic to her tribe. She walks the walk and talks the talk.

Stage 5: What looks different in the world for you right now?
I track my macros. I have learnt to be true to myself and do not allow people pleasing to control my journey. I can pull myself up and have stopped sabotaging my own results.

Stage 6: What challenges have you faced?
I have faced other people's judgements. I choose not to drink because I'd rather eat food than waste my macros on alcohol. People assume I can't have fun because of that. I prove them wrong. I have been challenged to be organised having a little one. I've had to step up and stand in my space with family and manage their expectations at family gatherings of what I should or should not eat. Sometimes my family can be classed as chocolate friends. I do cop a little bit of flak from them for not always indulging in unhealthy foods. In saying that I can make hot chips fit, which is my favourite.

What has your mentor taught you?
People pleasing is not healthy and is a way of outsourcing your self-worth. It's not a useful strategy for being true to yourself. Crash diets mess with your hormones and impact your fertility.

Stage 7: What do you need to face to be the hero of your own journey?
As a mother, getting back on track was scary. Mum guilt is a real thing. By putting myself first, I felt like I was neglecting my son. But really, I wasn't as I knew deep down that if I gave to myself first then I would be a better mother for him. I have wonderful strawberry friends that support me on this journey. Now I realise that chocolate friends do not understand and will just pass their judgement anyway.

Stage 8: What ordeals have you faced?
Being a mum you have a little one to care for and put first. Being out of balance and overcoming the fear of others judging me as a mum.

Stage 9: How were they life changing?
They made me stronger mentally and helped me push through another barrier. I put myself first and pulled myself up on the excuses like I have no time and a baby.

What tools and resources do you have now that are unbreakable?
I am not afraid to ask for help so I can have me time. I'm more adaptable, as I was always someone who trained in the morning now I have to train in the evening.

What looks different in this world for you right now?
Balance and flexibility.

Sasha is at stage 10 where she is going to use all her skills, tools, strategies and everything Empowered Eating has taught her to step onto the sports modelling stage and the powerlifting platform. She will model to her son strength, resilience and health. This will be her legacy.

Do you want to uplevel even further?

Think of movies or books that follow the hero's journey. How do they follow this formula in their story? *Harry Potter, The Lion King, Matrix, Lord of the Rings, Aladdin* and *Spiderman* all follow the exact steps outlined above. Marco Polo, Victoria Woodhull (the first female to speak before congress) and Malala are real-life examples. Can you think of any others? Could they be your models of excellence? Find someone who has gone on the journey before you and model their behaviour.

Questions from Empowered Eating clients just like you

What if I can't decide where I am at?
Start by filling out each of the questions and this will give you a clearer understanding.

Can you have several examples of where you are on the hero's journey?
You may wish to write the hero's journey for your career and then compartmentalise by doing it for your personal life. For example, my client Trish was able to map across everything in her career to a completed journey as she is retired yet when it comes to her fitness journey, she is only at stage 4.

Strategies for your Empowered Eating Toolbox

1. By mapping your journey into the hero's journey it will enable you to have peace that you are moving towards your goal and that it is possible, even with setbacks. Most of us get stuck because we don't see everything, just what is happening in front of us. By completing this task you can inject hope and take pride in how far you have come.

2. By following the hero's journey, you become hyperaware of what might be next, enabling you to tap into your intuition and look for signs. I hope this book was a sign to show you anything is possible. Just like the stories I share in this book from my clients, you too can take the next step towards having a life that you deserve.

3. If you have almost completed a hero's journey in your life, it may be the nudge you need to take the next step in leaving a legacy. Like my client who got herself out of $30,000 of debt and is now going to write a book on money mindset. It is her calling to impact the world.

Chapter 12

Piranha to nirvana

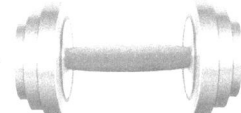

Whatever the mind can conceive and believe, the mind can achieve.

Napoleon Hill

To set yourself free from emotional eating you need a compelling enough vision to pull you. To do this we are going to write a creative writing piece about your future 12 months from now.

We sabotage our results when we feel unsafe. As human beings we like to return to the familiar. If you cannot envision what your life will be like at your ideal body weight then you are going to return to your previous shape. This is why I prep my clients for photoshoots. They then have physical documentation of their new normal and are less likely to return to their familiar world. They become familiar with the unfamiliar. Another way of doing that is to create a creative writing piece about your future.

As Jack Canfield says:

> Elite athletes use it. The super-rich use it. And peak performers in all fields now use it. That power is called visualisation. The daily practice of visualising your dreams as already complete can rapidly accelerate your achievement of those dreams, goals and ambitions.

Steve Nash has a 90.4% success rate for his free throw in basketball because of visualisation. It primes his brain and body for the upcoming motor skills. Like Steve, through this exercise we are going to prime your brain and body for success in your life. You will be programmed to accept the unfamiliar and make it familiar.

If it seems all a little too woo-woo, think how the placebo effect works. Science has proven that the mind is powerful beyond our comprehension. Let's use that power for your journey to success.

Remember the reticular activating system (RAS)? By writing this piece, it gives the mind something to focus on. Right this minute think of what your hand is feeling? Maybe this book? Maybe you are reading from a kindle and you can feel the plastic? You might feel cold, you might feel warm. You weren't conscious of that before I mentioned it. The RAS will focus on whatever you turn your attention towards.

Before anything is created it must be imagined in the mind. Think of the humble light bulb. Thomas Edison imagined it first before he actually created it. Visualisation works because:

- It increases motivation and a reason to strengthen your resilience muscle

- Daydreaming creates happy endorphins running around in your body
- By reading this journal piece every day you will create stronger emotional bonds to your dreams which means you will be able to dig deep when things get hard.

Ask yourself: have I created enough of a compelling reason why yet?

See yourself as you choose to be

Every year I write a journal piece called, 'See yourself as you choose to be'. It's a snapshot of a future time. I have evidence THIS WORKS!

I wrote one in Dec 2014 as a visualisation activity that dreamed 2015 into life. I doubled my business income, achieved 18% body fat, broke commonwealth records, saw my family four times in the year, developed spiritually, attracted a dark featured man (who in 2019 become my husband), crossed things off my bucket list, travelled and so much more because I set the intention. *I dreamt my husband and so much more into my life.*

I did it again for 2017. I was outsourced for motivational speaking, took silver at Worlds, went to Greece, made an impact on the world with my videos, consistently trained 30 clients, took Fridays as my study day, saved 20k for my holiday, studied another NLP course and had grown spiritually.

I did it again for 2018. Got engaged, fourth at Worlds, broke Commonwealth and Australian records in 110kg bench, started regular seminars, studied another NLP course, uplevelled my friends, put ladies on stage and the platform, travelled to Europe.

To me this is part of my goal setting, how I design my life and how I get things done. Visualisation is a very powerful tool, and more so when attached to emotions and feelings.

Visualising your goals and desires activates your creative subconscious so you can start generating ideas to achieve your goal. It also programs your brain (and your RAS) to more easily perceive and recognise what you need, and through the law of attraction, you will begin to draw the people, resources and circumstances into your life that will help you along the way. And importantly, it provides you with motivation to do what it takes to make your dreams a reality.

Activity

To provide inspiration for this creative writing piece start with the wheel of life and rate where you are in each part of your life. Then imagine it is New Year's Eve of the following year and you're are looking back on the year. Talk about all the things that you have achieved, the crazy things you've tried, the impact you have made on the world, the relationships that have strengthened.

To increase those creative juices answer the following questions:

Who will you spend time with?

_____

What will your day look like?

_____

How much money will you have in the bank?

_____

What do your personal relationships look like? Family, partner?

_____

What position will you hold at work?

_____

How will you give back?

_____

What will you do in your free time?

_____

How will you grow spiritually?

_____

What books will you read?

_____

What talents will you develop?

_____

What friendships will you nurture?

_____

What does family time look like?

_____

How will you grow closer to your significant other?

_____

What will your date nights look like?

_____

What debt have you removed from your life?

_____

How much is in your emergency account?

_____

What do you need to do health-wise?

_____

How often will you see the doctor, dentist or get a massage?

_____

Who will support you on your health journey?

_____

What will your body composition look like?

_____

What does your morning routine look like?

_____

What will your house look like?

_____

What do you need to get organised?

_____

How will you give to your soul?

_____

What getaways will you take?

_____

How do you feel energy wise?

_____

When you are present what do you feel, see, hear?

_____

What's the one place you have always wanted to go to?

_____

How will you live by example for other people?

_____

What lights you up?

_____

What will you learn?

_____

Do you want to uplevel even further?

To take this to the next level you can add images to your vison board that we mentioned in Chapter 1. Vision boards can be images and photos cut out and stuck to a canvas or corkboard. I have also used a magnetic whiteboard as this enabled me to write quotes, mantras and specific targets with a marker. You can use scrapbooking materials, glitter, stickers and paint. Images can be printed from the internet, Pinterest or cut from magazines. Get creative and have fun! Once completed this becomes a super power to activate the RAS. Where are you going to hang it? Mine is in my office as I am in there every day. It could be in your bedroom so you see it every morning when you wake. If it's small enough then inside your pantry door is a great place. Maybe create two, one for your bedroom and one for the pantry door.

Questions from Empowered Eating clients just like you

What if I can't write?
The only person reading this is you so don't worry about spelling mistakes, grammar and punctuation. Just let it flow and be creative. You might write several pages, then, in a day or two, come back to it.

I'm stuck for inspiration...
Pinterest is great for creating boards of your dreams especially if you are a visual person.

I can't get in the mood.
I find that laying on my tummy (tummy time) allows me to be in that daydream state that allows my dreams to flow out of me.

Strategies for your Empowered Eating Toolbox

1. Read this journal piece every day as a reminder of what you are working toward, creating strong imagery to pull you out of the cycle of bingeing.

2. Look for signs, opportunities and action steps that you can take to get you closer to your goals.

3. Find ways to bring this image to life. Do you need to go test drive that new car, stand on the stage that you want to present at, go to the open house in your favourite suburb, go to the travel agent to talk about your holiday, buy that hot dress you want to wear to next year's Christmas party. Anything to make this tangible and real.

Afterword

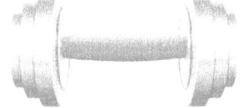

I'm so proud of you for getting through this book. I truly hope that you have found it empowering. You have all the tools you need to succeed and I am here to give you permission to go after the life that you deserve. It isn't going to be easy, the unsexiest advice I can give you is 'do the work'. I know that isn't what you wanted to hear – but I am telling you *it is the only way*. Do each of the exercises, go to those deep dark places. Only then does a phoenix rise from the ashes. You can and you will rise strong.

Those of us who binge eat continue to get in our own way. Over and over again we get close to change, but we feel too unsafe to stay there. Even my most committed transformation clients at one point have slipped up. I like to use the analogy of quitting smoking. I smoked from the ages of 16 to 21, I started because I wanted to be cool and as you remember, I was bullied for being little miss goody two shoes. When I first quit I would go to parties and have the occasional cigarette. Eventually I could get through a whole party without a cigarette. Fifteen plus years later, I'm not a smoker. However, if I had used each of those slip ups as a reason to keep smoking I would be sitting here with a terrible smoker's cough, dry wrinkly skin and a disrespect for my body.

You have a choice. YOU are the only person who is responsible for taking the first step and starting the journey back to being SEXY, CONFIDENT and LOVED inside and out. You deserve to learn to stand up for your own happiness and glow from the inside out.

About the Author

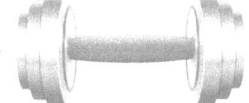

To touch, move and inspire women to have an empowered relationship with food, so that they can be free to have the life they deserve. To help them become better partners, mothers and career women and make an impact on their community.

This is the driving force behind this book.

Kim has lived this journey herself, and through her experience and professional knowledge she shows you how to have a more empowered relationship with food, your partner, your children and the people you work with. These tools and strategies come from her own life, client coaching sessions and a never-ending quest to learn better ways to empower people.

Since starting her career in 2006, Kim has had a deep-seated passion to help people like you be the best version of themselves and create the life they truly deserve. To have long-term success you need to focus on the trifecta: training, nutrition and most important (yet least considered) the mind.

Kim is a qualified personal trainer, Recomp body composition re-composer, neuro-linguistic programming practitioner, life coach, strength and conditioning trainer and rehab trainer.

Currently the holder of multiple Australian, Commonwealth and Oceania records, she has represented Australia at an international level since 2014, including a gold medal at the Commonwealth Games and silver at the World Powerlifting Championships. With a background in competitive bodybuilding, running half marathons and gymnastics, her love of powerlifting is evident and backs up the belief that it makes you strong from the inside out... and that you'll look great in heels (Kim's other love).

A few words from the author herself:

I have a philosophy that I encourage clients to adopt which is to nurture soul time. For me that is spending time with my husband, grounding myself in prayer and meditation, walking my blue heeler Delta, reading a book with Tashka the Russian blue and going to the beach to feel the sun on my back while watching the waves crash. I grew up in Noosa on the Sunshine Coast so salt is in my blood. I may live far from the beach in Canberra now, but the drive to Coogee gives me an opportunity to listen to an audiobook on personal development. This is my favourite way to learn. I have a saying, 'My brain is worth too much money not to invest in learning'.

I have hit rock bottom myself, bingeing out of control to deal with stress and unresolved issues. I grew up in domestic violence, my biological father left when I was two, my ex-boyfriend committed suicide, I was subjected to a horrendous crime, grew up without a father to protect me and used food to cope and control. I don't tell you this for sympathy as I have rewritten what my past means to me. I tell you these tragedies as a way to give you hope. Hope that you can change your future. You CAN rewrite your past; you CAN rewrite what it means to you. Your past doesn't need to poison your future.

ABOUT THE AUTHOR

Bingeing doesn't have to be the only way you cope. I have been binge-free since 2010 because I invested in a coach who helped me. Now it is my turn to help you. This is your journey, you deserve to be free. You are the expert in your own life, my only job is to empower you with the right tools and strategies. I have the knowledge, education and the drive to get you there. Are you ready to work? Do you give yourself permission?

- https://www.facebook.com/Transformations-by-Kim-234947206582487/
- https://www.instagram.com/kim.stevenson.farmakis
- https://www.linkedin.com/in/kim-stevenson-farmakis-2b6b68bb
- https://transformationsbykim.com/home

Acknowledgements

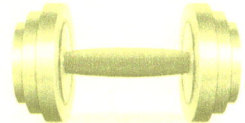

There are many great books that I have read over the years and a few are mentioned throughout this book. I would like to thank these authors for their valuable insights into human behaviour. In particular:

The 5 Love Languages, Garry Chapman (Strand Publishing, 1992)

The Hero with A Thousand Faces, Joseph Campbell (New World Publishing, 1949)

Awaken the Giant Within, Tony Robbins (Simon & Schuster, 1991)

Elegantly Simple Solutions to Complex People Problems, Jaemin Frazer (Jaemin Frazer and Associates, 2018)

Get Rich, Lucky Bitch! Denise Duffield Thomas (Hay House UK Ltd, 2018)

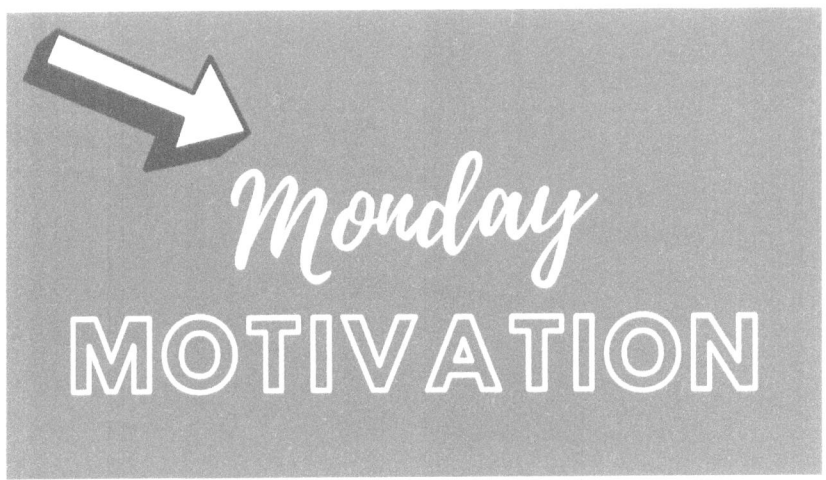

Loved the book and want more strategies?

I want you to be confident and have a healthy relationship with food. This means continually doing the inner work that is easy to ignore. To help you to keep facing your food demons subscribe to receive a powerful 5-minute video straight to your inbox each week, with proven tools and strategies that work.

https://transformationsbykim.com/home

Simply click [GET YOUR MONDAY MOTIVATION] and you're all set!

And if you haven't already downloaded your book bonuses, head to https://transformationsbykim.com/bookbonuses to receive your special gifts.

KIM STEVENSON FARMAKIS

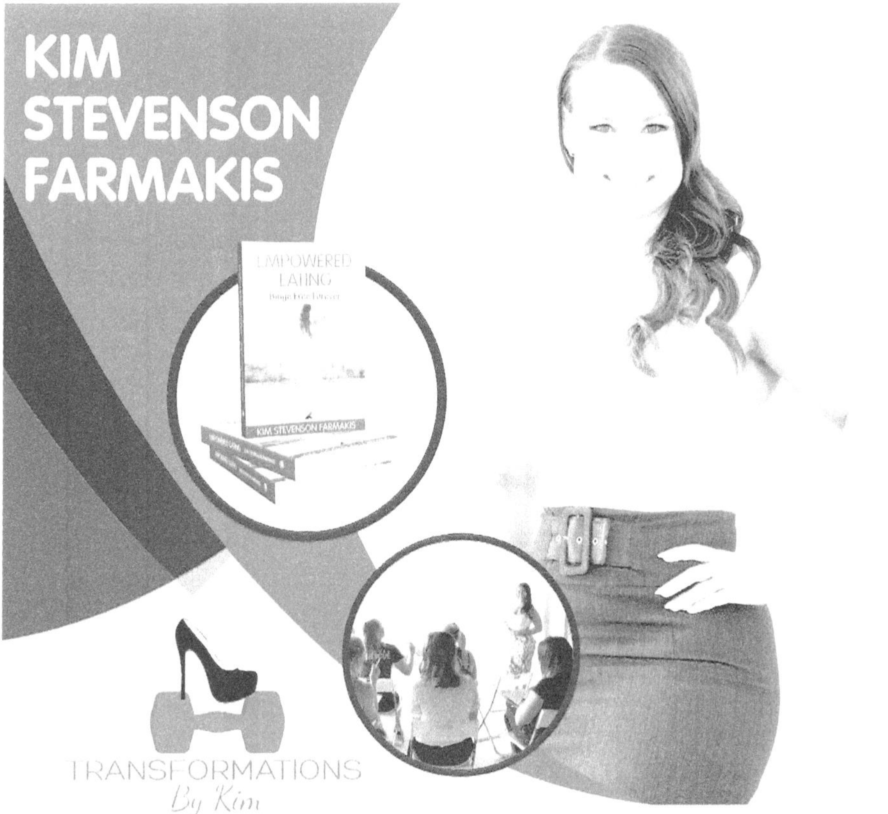

TRANSFORMATIONS By Kim

Do you have a podcast or publication? Are you organising a seminar or conference?

Kim is highly sought after as a speaker and has contributed to various media including Body and Soul magazine, ABC radio, the Jaemin Frazer Podcast and Canberra Times. She shared her insights on empowered eating for the Fernwood Wellness Challenge and is a regular speaker at gyms throughout Canberra and beyond.

In her energetic and engaging presentations, Kim shares the mindset tools she used to recover from an eating disorder, traumatic childhood and a destructive perfectionist all or nothing mentality. These breakthroughs enabled her to take silver at the World Powerlifting Championships, bench 117.5kgs at only 63kgs body weight and break numerous Commonwealth and Australian records. Her story will inspire your attendees!

The key takeaways include:

Empowered mindset
- Why fear drives us and where does it come from
- How to overcome fears and limiting beliefs
- How to overcome obstacles and identify triggers
- How to develop your self-love and confidence
- How to deal with all types of rejection
- The neuroscience of success
- How to inspire change

Life lessons women can learn from strength training
- How failing faster under the bar gives you success in the boardroom
- Facing your demons when training and in life
- How to succeed at the game of life outside of training

Secrets to success in weight loss and life
- How to find the right mentor so you don't waste your hard-earned money
- How to supercharge your goal setting
- Why motivation doesn't work
- Conquering your past so you don't sabotage your results
- Powerful steps to overcome emotional eating

Since 2006, Kim has specialised in binge/emotional eating and strength and conditioning coaching, helping hundreds of clients achieve their goals. She has the knowledge, experience and strategies to educate your audience and give them the tools they need to align their mindset with their goals and feel empowered!

The Canberra Times   **The Chronicle**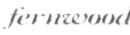

To find out more or make a booking, get in touch:
www.transformationsbykim.com/contact

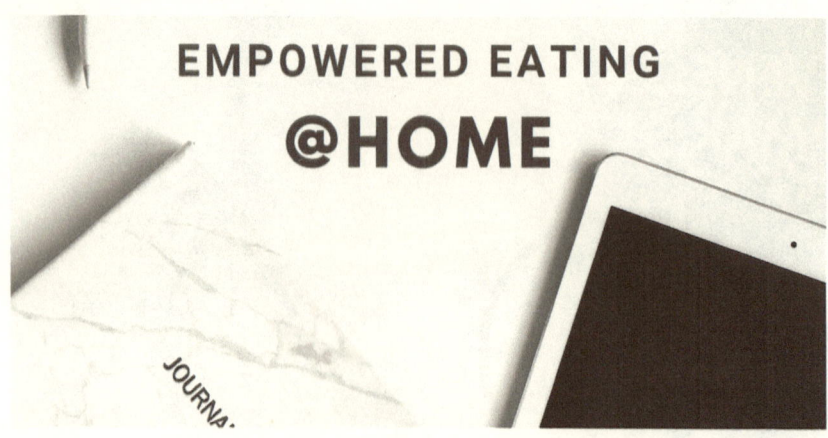

Have you ever felt out of control with food? Are you stuck on the diet merry-go-round and lack the confidence to get off? Then the EMPOWERED EATING AT HOME PROGRAM IS FOR YOU!

Presented by life coach, emotional eating specialist and international-level powerlifter Kim Stevenson, this program will give you the tools and support you need to overcome your emotional eating and take control once and for all.

Aligned with weekly group coaching sessions on Skype hosted by Kim, the program teaches you the principles of empowered eating and includes positive anchors to propel your growth. You'll get lifetime membership to resources and ongoing access to the Facebook support group for accountability and support.

Through proven NLP and life coaching strategies, coaching videos and worksheets with tools you can practise now you'll learn how to:

- ✓ Master your emotions so that you are in control, not food

- ✓ Find that confident woman before the yo-yo dieting and weight gain

EMPOWERED EATING
@HOME

- ✓ Be sexy from every fibre of your soul so you can wear whatever you want

- ✓ Educate yourself and have a healthy relationship with food for life

- ✓ Break the cycle, stop eating emotions and be consistent

- ✓ Find out why you sabotage own success from an unconscious level

- ✓ Live full to your full potential and finally be happy

All videos are available immediately so there is no need to wait – you can get started now!

Click [Empowered Eating @Home] to start your journey today. https://transformationsbykim.com/

Looking forward to working with you!

Dare to Dream

Kim Stevenson

Notes

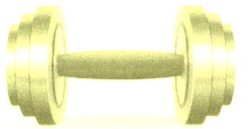

www.ingramcontent.com/pod-product-compliance
Lightning Source LLC
Chambersburg PA
CBHW021149080526
44588CB00008B/274